Healing Rosacea

WITH ANTI-INFLAMMATORY DIET
AND HEALTHY LIFESTYLE

WITHOUT USING MEDICATION

WRITTEN BY ALICIA PIOT

TEXT EDITTED BY ALLY MITCHELL

Copyright Notice

COPYRIGHT 2023 ALICIA PIOT

All rights reserved. No part of this book may be used or reproduced by any means, graphic, electronic, or mechanical, including photocopying, recording, taping, or by any information storage retrieval system, without the written permission of the publisher except in the case of brief quotations embodied in critical articles and reviews.

This book details the author's personal experiences with and opinions about rosacea, chronic inflammation and general health. The author is not a healthcare provider and this book is not intended to be a substitute for the medical advice of a licensed physician. The reader should consult with their doctor in any matters relating to his/her health.

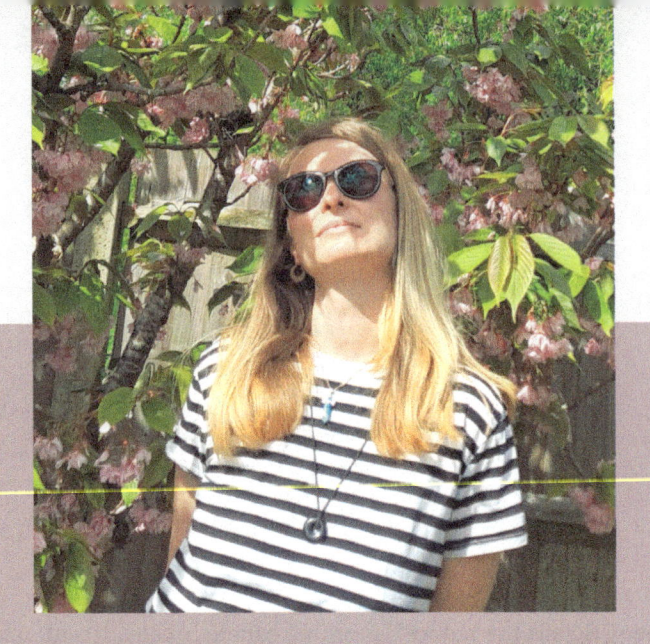

Hey there, I'm Alicia

I'm a former rosacea sufferer, who managed to reverse her skin condition using healthy, natural methods and without taking any medication. It's been nearly three years now since I'm rosacea free.

I'm here to share my rosacea healing journey- all the changes I implemented in my life which enabled me to heal my rosacea and maintain my now clear and inflammation-free skin. I truly believe my story and my advice can help you if you struggle with this condition. I hope we can take the first steps together in order to nurture your health and heal your skin.

In this book, I will talk about all my steps to healthy, inflammation-free skin. Yet, I want to assure you, I will not be recommending any miracle medication, treatment, one-week solution or a particular food that will clear your skin instantly.

Yes, I know we are bombarded with commercials and paid recommendations of "astonishing-results" rosacea treatments, lasers, derma cosmetics, etc. Guess what, I've tried most of them and nothing worked.

Today, after nearly three years of clear skin, I know that any quick fix for rosacea must be complete nonsense. There is no product, facial treatment, ingredient, magical supplement or even medication that can heal your skin. The origins of skin inflammatory conditions (rosacea being one of them) are very complex. To defeat them we need to concentrate on the roots of the problem and fix them right where they initiate. With this book, I would like to indicate to you all the layers that need your attention in order to get to grips with rosacea.

It took me around six months to completely clear my skin – from the moment I decided to tackle this problem, learn about my body and follow my gut instinct. I took a natural, holistic and very intuitive approach toward my body and I must say, it worked wonders. My rosacea healing journey included endless research, reading numerous medical articles and books, analysing many studies, but also listening to stories of other rosacea sufferers and finally learning to listen to my own body.

This healing journey had many ups and downs, I took many steps forward and sometimes steps back. But eventually, my rosacea reversed and it was an amazing reward after many months of determination, focus and consistency. But the best reward for me now is the understanding of what my body needs to be happy, healthy and in balance. This is all thanks to my experience with rosacea.

This book is created with the intention to guide you through the complexity of inflammatory skin conditions but also to give you an idea of the steps which you can take to reverse your rosacea. I hope you are ready to take this journey with me. And yes, I have many important lessons to share but please remember: you are the only person who can fix your skin, by listening to your body and, day by day, by making the right choices for your health.

BEFORE WE START, I WOULD LIKE TO ENCOURAGE YOU TO:

- carry out your own extensive research on rosacea
- think deeper than just your skin
- explore each hypothesis I mention in this book
- keep reading
- and most importantly, listen to your gut instinct because deep down we know what is best for us and how to solve all our problems

TABLE OF
Contents

01. The beginning of my rosacea journey — 01
How it all started for me. How I knew right away that I had rosacea. How I felt about it. What the doctors advised me and why I didn't want to listen to them;

02. Reading the signs — 08
How I started figuring out the truth behind rosacea: is it just a skin condition or is it a symptom of something else?

03. Realising how to approach rosacea — 12
All about the break-through thoughts, theories and suppositions that made me realise how I can reverse my rosacea; learning about chronic inflammation;

04. Gut health and rosacea — 19
What can be potentially going on with your gut health that caused you to develop rosacea?

05. Liver health and rosacea — 25
About optimal liver function and its connection with chronic skin conditions;

06. Do Demodex mites cause rosacea? — 28
What's the easy way to find out?

07. Time to reflect- what caused my rosacea — 30
Let's see if you can relate...

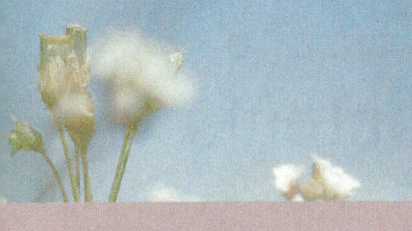

TABLE OF
Contents

08. Rosacea healing diets — 35
The right nutrition is a crucial step for reversing rosacea...

09. Stress management and emotional wellbeing — 78
The second most crucial step after diet;

10. Healthy sleep pattern — 89
Why good sleep is so important for healing rosacea;

11. Sensible approach to over-the-counter medication and antibiotics — 91
Why taking regularly over-the-counter medication can contribute to your skin inflammation;

12. Physical activity and rosacea — 93
How can moving your body help with rosacea;

13. Rosacea skincare — 96
We are bombarded with rosacea targeting products everywhere, no wonder we can get confused...

14. The summary of my rosacea healing journey — 101
And some gentle advice for you!

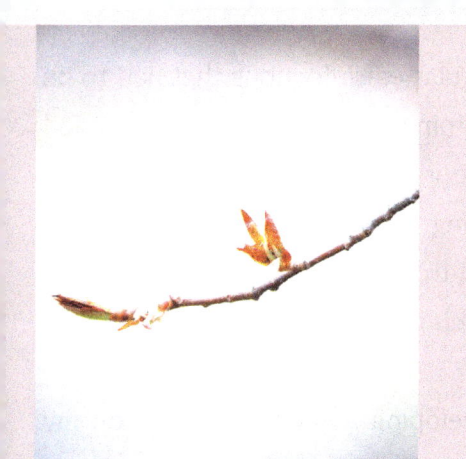

01

The beginning of my rosacea journey

To start, I must say: I never had perfect skin. When I was a teenager, I used to struggle with teen acne, then in my early twenties, I was diagnosed with hormonal acne (large, painful pimples on my chin). My skin settled down after I had my first child at the age of 26. I would have occasional breakouts after I became a mother, but nothing major.

Four years later, I had my second child. During the pregnancy and for the first year after giving birth, my skin was in good condition. But throughout breastfeeding, I would regularly get mastitis, an infection of the milk glands which not only makes the breast incredibly painful, but also causes flu-like symptoms – fever, body aches and chills. Generally, you feel very unwell. I was desperate to breastfeed as long as I could as I always believed long-term breastfeeding gives countless benefits to children's health. I breastfed my first child for two and a half years and I wanted to do the same with my youngest. But the breasts gland infection kept coming back, and every time, I was prescribed antibiotics.

On top of that I was having regular ear infections that had to be treated with antibiotics too. Within a period of just over a year, I believe I took eight or nine courses of antibiotics. Eventually, after 14 months of breastfeeding, I had to give up. Meanwhile, that time was also complicated by problems in my relationship. There was a lot going on and I felt permanently distressed.

During that time, I started developing a small red patch on my left cheek. I didn't really think much of it at first as it was easy enough to cover up with make-up. One month later, a few spots appeared on the red patch. As a busy mum with small children and dealing with relationship problems, a little redness and breakout was the last thing on my mind. I decided to use some of the acne fighting products which had worked for me in the past. But this time they didn't help; instead I felt like all those products were making it worse. One month later my left cheek was looking terrible. It felt hot, painful and inflamed. By then I knew I had rosacea.

How? I already knew a few people with this particular skin condition. My dad was one of them. He had been suffering from rosacea for the last 15 years and it had been a nightmare for him. At first, he was prescribed a variety of steroid creams, then antibiotic cream. All of them just worsened his skin. Then he took oral antibiotics. I remember his skin would improve after a while, but when he stopped taking the antibiotic, the rosacea came back. At some point, even his eyelids were affected. I remember how insecure he felt, how much he suffered, how much money he spent trying to sort his skin out.

My dad never gained full control over his skin and eventually gave up trying any another treatments. Within those 15 years he fluctuated with slightly better skin and moments of severity. He didn't have a clue what aggravated the condition and why it sometimes settled. It was like a lottery, who knew what the next month would bring... Throughout the years, he learnt to live with it, and in a way, accepted his skin as it was.

When my own face started to resemble my dad's at its worst, my concern grew so I went to the doctor. As soon as he saw me his diagnosis was clear and concrete: "You have rosacea. I am sorry," he said.
I knew exactly why he added "I am sorry".
"Rosacea is chronic and incurable..." I said.
"Yes," he confirmed, "have you heard about rosacea before?"
"I have," I said. "My dad has it and one of my friends had it for a long time."
"Oh, your dad has it?"
"Yes, do you think genetics can play a role here?"
"It is not really known for sure, but we do observe some inherited tendencies," he said.

At this point a wave of hopelessness came over me. If it was genetic, I would have no chance of having a "normal" looking face ever again, I thought. In my mind I could picture my dad's skin and every battle he undertook until finally giving up. Was this my future as well?

I never had perfect skin (who does?) and I was ok with that. But I'd also never had such a bad, inflamed and red complexion.

I didn't ever like using much make-up; I didn't feel myself with a full face of products. But I definitely didn't feel myself with red, inflamed and spotty skin either...

There is a big difference between how you think you would cope with bad skin hypothetically and how much it can actually affect your life when you are facing the problem. I was very lucky to have been brought up by a confident woman, my mum, who would never prioritise her looks. My mum was always very relaxed about her appearance, and I think I turned out much like her. I would never be too concerned about my looks. I could go anywhere without make-up and wearing joggers and I was always comfortable within myself.

But rosacea changed this. Most of the time, my mind was occupied by my bad skin, completely removing my confidence. I become obsessed with it. I would look in the mirror 50 times a day, worrying it was getting worse. I would buy tonnes of make-up products in the attempt to cover it up, but nothing helped and my skin never looked good. I also felt like I had to explain to every single person I came across why my skin looked so bad. I started spending most of my time researching, reading and watching videos of people sharing their rosacea stories. Of course, I was drawn to the stories of miraculous rosacea cures. Influenced by all the stories, I spent vast sums of money on various rosacea products and treatments; I even purchased an expensive LED mask for home use. None of the products made any difference to my skin. Yes, one day it would seem better, then it would become inflamed. But I couldn't see any relation to the products I was using.

Even though I felt desperate, I was resistant to trying antibiotics, steroids and Accutane. Why? Because none of them had worked for my dad. I also have a friend who, before I met her, had suffered from really bad rosacea and she had taken antibiotics for six months in order to clear it. Yes, her skin improved but she started having serious gut problems and soon after, was diagnosed with Crohn's disease. Now she believes there is a link between her long antibiotic use with her bowel disorder. When I hear various rosacea battle stories, people reveal that the result of medications were only temporary, and later the rosacea returned with ferocity.

This turned out to be a recurring theme, a common experience for many rosacea sufferers to be disillusioned by medications and treatments. I simply knew I was not going to go down that path and take antibiotics, steroid creams or isotretinoin (Accutane or Roaccutane). No chance, I thought, I am wise enough to learn from other people's experiences. Meanwhile, I had seen four different doctors, my GP and three private dermatologists. One of them advised me to use Soolanta cream, which fights Demodex mites; I tried it for several weeks but didn't notice any improvement, quite the opposite. Eventually all the doctors I had seen gave me the same recommendations – oral antibiotics, steroid or antibiotic creams and if these didn't show results, isotretinoin. One dermatologist was also advising me a series of rosacea laser treatments.

This all made me feel resentful and hopeless. They must have known what they are prescribing and advising wouldn't solve the core of my problem, just suppress the symptoms for a while.

When I look back at that time, I am very disappointed that not a single doctor even asked me about my diet or lifestyle, nobody tried to look for the cause of my skin chronic inflammation.

And don't get me wrong, I am not saying you must dismiss your doctor's advice. Of course it's up to you what path you decide to take with regard to your rosacea treatment. Personally, I have noticed when it comes to skin conditions, conventional medicine seems to be failing because it only focuses on the superficial level, on treating the symptoms instead of the root cause. Back then, I already knew the conventional medical approach wouldn't help me. I would not be satisfied with a short-term fix.

I wanted to discover the real reason behind my skin issues and find the long-term solution. To me, it felt like the doctors I had seen didn't really want to help me.

They didn't appear to have any interest in:
- Why has my skin been reacting this way?
- What is the core of the problem?
- How to solve the problem at its core?

At that point, I hadn't started my extensive research, but I already understood that if we only suppress the body's reactions, the problem will still exist and all we do is cover it up. Until we eliminate the reason, our problem will come back sooner or later. There are countless stories of rosacea sufferers taking antibiotics, isotretinoin or using steroid creams for a long time but without any positive results. Sometimes these meds don't work at all. Often they are temporary solutions, then when people finish their treatments, boom – rosacea comes back, often much more severely.

It's been over four years since my journey with rosacea first began but it still feels to me like conventional medicine is failing to treat this skin condition so they make us believe that it is chronic, we have to live with it; all we can do is alleviate the symptoms.

Intuitively, I didn't agree with this approach back when I first developed rosacea symptoms and I definitely don't agree with it now. As for today I am one of the many examples that **rosacea is fully reversible...**

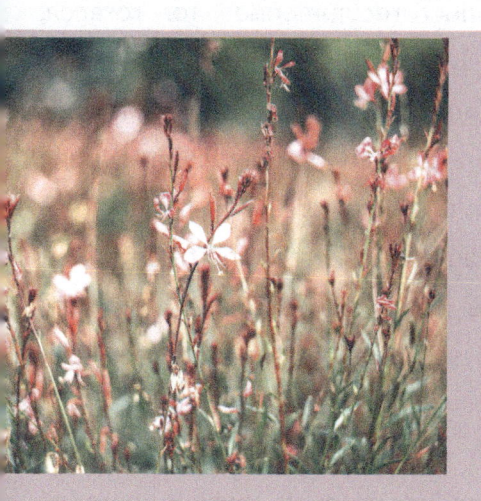

"Medication used for rosacea only suppresses the body's reactions. The problem will still exist. All we do is cover it up. Until we eliminate the reason, our problem will come back sooner or later."

ALICIA PIOT

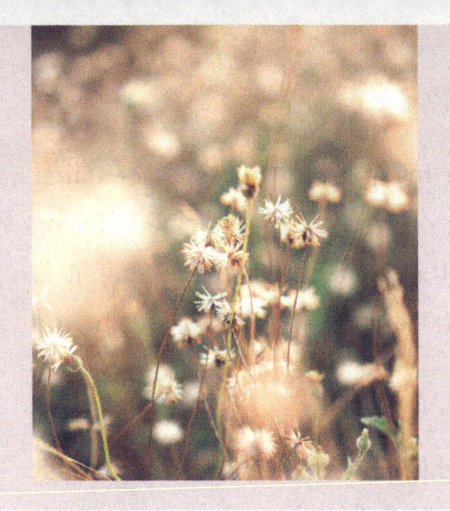

02

Reading the signs

Six months of rosacea madness was enough for me. It was getting worse and worse every day, to the point that make up couldn't cover it anymore and I didn't want to leave the house as I was so embarrassed of my skin. I stopped attending my art classes and I was avoiding all social contact. I kept spending money on every single product recommended for rosacea, anything with good reviews. I spent all my free time reading about rosacea and watching YouTube videos with tips on how to fight it; I truly had become obsessed. Luckily, I had young children at the time so I couldn't fully immerse myself in my new 'passion'. But believe me, the amount of stress and frustration it cost me to even look in the mirror, the extremely low self-esteem that came with it, self-blaming and self-hate, the constant agitation.

I kept trying numerous 'wonder' products (which were so expensive!), face treatments and LED masks that supposedly reduced redness. On top of that I tried tonnes of foundations and concealers to try to hide the spots and redness.

I stopped eating spicy foods, nightshades (including tomatoes, potatoes, bell peppers) which many people recommended. And you know what? Nothing, nothing made a difference. Months were passing and my frustration was growing; I felt so hopeless. Soon my mood was deeply affected and I reached a low point where rosacea was impacting all aspects of my life – my family, my relationship with my partner, my social life, my daily motivation.

Thinking back on that now, I can't understand why I took it so seriously. I am an intelligent person with lots of passions, and I have never concentrated that much on my appearance, clothes or make up. Why did I care so much? Why did I allow the red skin make me feel so low?

But one day I woke up and I thought: "enough." Rosacea is a skin condition, but it was affecting more than my skin. The redness and spots were truly affecting my wellbeing... I couldn't carry on as I was. I knew I was not going to accept it. I really wanted to heal. And as I became clear about my intention, things finally started to take a new direction...

One day I came across a podcast about all sorts of chronic skin conditions by Dr Mark Adam Hyman, an American physician, well-recognised in the wellness world as an advocate for functional medicine. In the podcast he voiced something I had been suspecting for a long time: a skin condition like rosacea, eczema, psoriasis, dermatitis or acne, are manifestations of some kind of systematic imbalance and abnormality. This theory really caught my attention as it was corresponding with my gut instinct regarding rosacea. Following this podcast, I searched for more information – causes and treatments according to functional medicine practitioners. I had finally found a ray of hope in my battle with rosacea...

I had spent months trying to beat the inflammation in my skin, and it had made no difference. Not just me, but my dad, my friend, people I follow on social media. We all had been focusing on our skin problems, still unable to solve it. But now I had found a whole new world of professionals, studies and evidence showing that the problem starts much deeper and thanks to functional medicine and supported by extended research, I could discover the most common and probable causes of rosacea.

After many months of failed attempts, this new perspective hit me like a lightening bolt and finally things started making sense to me. I was able to put all the pieces of the puzzle together: my dad's and friend's rosacea experiences, online stories from rosacea sufferers, my own defeat. Now, I started to look at rosacea from a different position- this condition wasn't my enemy anymore, it was a

Functional medicine (FM) is a holistic and patient-centred approach to health and is based on science and evolving research. Functional medicine always looks for the reason for illness to occur rather than treating or suppressing the symptoms. FM practitioners point out that the same symptom, for example, depression, can be caused by many different factors and underlying health issues therefore long-lasting health benefits can come from identifying and addressing the root cause. **FM focuses on a patient's individual circumstances like genes, environment, diet and lifestyle in order to determine the potential cause behind the condition and to establish a personalised treatment plan.**

message sent from my body that it's struggling with some internal issues. I was extremely curious to know more, to discover my rosacea underlying causes and I began to nurture the general topic of skin inflammatory conditions.

Day by day, the feeling of hopelessness lessened and the confidence that I could actually 'fix' my skin grew.

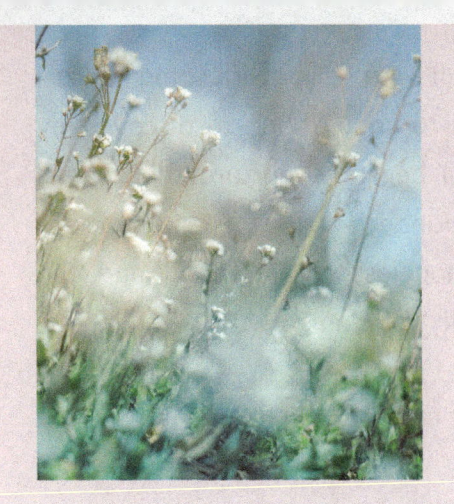

03
Realising how to approach rosacea

Let's start by understanding what rosacea is

Rosacea is recognised by the medical world as a chronic inflammatory skin condition. It's characteristics include persistent facial redness, pimples, swelling, and small, superficial dilated blood vessels. Mostly it affects the cheeks, nose, forehead and chin. Severe cases may bring about a red, enlarged nose or/and swollen eyelids. It is believed that rosacea affects mostly people with paler skin although nowadays rosacea occurs in all skin types. It is estimated to affect up to 10% of the world's population.

For decades, the cause of rosacea was labelled as unknown, and it used to be linked to genetic predispositions. Nowadays, the science and medical world is starting to link most chronic inflammatory conditions to inappropriate diets, lifestyles and gut dysfunctions.

Rosacea was once considered as an incurable skin condition. There are treatments available that may improve the symptoms but the results (if there were any at all) were usually short-term.

"Treatment is typically with metronidazole, doxycycline, minocycline, or tetracycline. When the eyes are affected, azithromycin eye drops may help. Other treatments with tentative benefit include brimonidine cream, ivermectin cream, and isotretinoin. Dermabrasion or laser surgery may also be used. The use of sunscreen is typically recommended."* Wikipedia

Because rosacea is so common nowadays, there are many ongoing studies researching this problem. When I started to learn about rosacea, I came across studies that were suggesting that it may be an outcome of systemic inflammation, for instance in the gut.

Those conclusions linking rosacea to systemic inflammation really resonated with me for a couple of reasons. My dad also struggled with digestion issues ever since I remember. My friend who suffered with severe rosacea was later diagnosed with Crohn's disease, an inflammatory bowel condition.

It also became clear to me as to why this condition wasn't curable. Conventional medicine concentrated on skin-level inflammation, making no difference to the real problem that lies internally. The medical treatments of antibiotics, steroids or creamed medications were not effective in the long-term because they only suppressed the symptoms rather than treating the cause.

Highlighting the above, I wouldn't like you to be alarmed or stressed that you have an underlying serious health issue. Rosacea, I believe, is a sign of a low-grade inflammation or imbalance in our bodies. There are people who suffer from rosacea for many years (like my dad). If anyone had severe underlaying conditions, the body would give them 'stronger' signals. My own tests (carried out by the NHS and privately) showed a mild inflammation in my gut.

Even though I wasn't feeling alarmed of any serious condition, I started to understand that my body was giving me a sign that there was some kind of imbalance or abnormality occurring in my system. To be fair, I sensed it right from the beginning but for a long time I was just suppressing that inner voice. All the doctors I had seen didn't seem to be too enthusiastic to refer me for any further tests as it was "only rosacea". I was disappointed, but at the same time I felt like I was being unreasonable not trusting the health authorities.

Thanks to functional medicine, its approach to skin conditions and all the studies behind it, I didn't feel irrational anymore. I wanted to discover the root cause of my skin problem and tackle it at its core. I started exploring general topics like inflammatory and chronic autoimmunological conditions, gut health, liver health and how it connected with each other. I was truly intrigued by my findings...

The first piece in the puzzle was to understand what inflammation and chronic inflammation are and the possible factors that cause them. I found so many eye opening articles and publications about all sorts of inflammatory conditions, so many inspiring podcasts, the list is endless. It all allowed me to get a wider perspective and I started to realise what had gone wrong in my own health, causing me to develop rosacea and what I needed to do to fix it...

What inflammation is and why it flares up in our bodies

Inflammation is a process in which the body fights against harmful infections, injuries or toxins, all in order to protect and heal itself.

When something damages our cells, our immune system's response is to release antibodies and proteins, increasing blood flow to the damaged area. For example, when we cut our skin, this process will last from a couple of hours, to a few days.

But when our bodies are in constant states of alert believing something bad is happening to the cells, we develop chronic inflammation.

Having our bodies in states of inflammation for a longer period of time may have a negative impact on our tissues and organs. All the studies suggest that long-term inflammation is a reason for many modern chronic conditions for example: Crohn's Disease, Ulcerative Colitis, Rheumatoid Arthritis, Psoriasis, Lupus, Asthma, Eczema, Rosacea, Hashimoto's disease, Insulin Resistance and many more. Most of these chronic diseases are believed to be rooted in low-grade inflammation that persists over a long period of time and goes unnoticed.

Medical studies also show that chronic inflammation is linked to the development of diseases like cancer, heart disease, type 2 diabetes, depression, cognitive decline and dementia (in older adults).

How is chronic inflammation diagnosed?

Certain blood tests can indicate that inflammation is occurring in our bodies. These tests include C-reactive protein (CRP) tests which indicate infections or inflammation in the general body (like the joints), and high-sensitivity C-reactive protein (hs-CRP) tests which reflect inflammation of the heart. Calprotectin stool tests measure if and how much inflammation is present in the intestines (bowels).

Often people don't even realise that they suffer from chronic inflammation. Sometimes it is not until they are diagnosed with one of the chronic inflammatory conditions.

Some common symptoms of chronic inflammation include chronic body pains, headaches, fatigue, depression or anxiety, gastrointestinal disorders (diarrhoea/constipation), unexplained weight gain or loss and frequent infections. These symptoms can vary between mild to severe and last for several months or years. Often symptoms are only subtle, so we don't think much about them because we have learnt to live with them. For many, it has become normal to use painkillers regularly to suppress the above symptoms.

If you experience any of the above symptoms repeatedly, the best idea is to speak to your doctor and arrange some tests.

What causes chronic inflammation?

Today many extensive studies take place searching for the causes of chronic inflammation. Researchers have been able to indicate several important reasons for prolonged occurrence of inflammation in the human body, and what is interesting is that the majority of those reasons are closely associated with the modern way of living:

- **No or too little physical activity.** When our muscles move, our bodies release anti-inflammatory chemicals into the bloodstream. People who don't meet the minimum physical activity recommendation have an increased risk of developing inflammatory diseases
- **Poor diet.** High in refined carbohydrates (sweets, cakes, alcohol, pastas, bread, pastries), low in fibre (fruits and vegetables), poor quality food due to mass farming practices, diets high in saturated fatty acids, higher Omega6 to Omega3 ratio, low in polyphenols, high in synthetic additives (like preservatives, flavor enrichments and colorants).
- **Smoking.** Is considered to be a major cause of chronic inflammation. Smoking cigarettes decreases the production of anti-inflammatory molecules and increases inflammation.
- **Prolonged psychological stress.** Studies show that chronic stress activates pro-inflammatory markers in the body.
- **Obesity.** Fat tissue, especially visceral fat (a deep layer of fat around the abdominal organs) produces pro-inflammatory chemicals.
- **Long-term exposure to industrial chemicals or polluted air.** Our bodies respond with inflammation to the toxins we absorb.

How is chronic inflammation treated?

There are some medications for chronic inflammation, but they are used to manage it – reduce inflammation and suppress symptoms – rather than cure or prevent it. For example, over-the-counter nonsteroidal anti-inflammatory drugs like aspirin and ibuprofen are often advised for relieving the symptoms of chronic inflammation like body aches and headaches (they are not advised when symptoms occur within the digestive tract).
Unfortunately long-term use of these medications is linked to an increased risk of several conditions, including peptic ulcer disease and kidney disease.

Another group of medications used for inflammatory conditions are steroids like Corticosteroids (a type of steroid hormone). They decrease inflammation and suppress the immune system. But again, long-term use of corticosteroids can lead to a variety of health complications like vision problems, high blood pressure, and osteoporosis.

Recent years have seen lots of discourse on long-term solutions to chronic inflammation. This focuses on making changes to modern lifestyles and diets that probably caused the chronic inflammation in the first place. I believe this discussion was first initiated by alternative health practitioners but as the extensive studies confirm its credibility, an increasing number of conventional medical doctors seem to be agreeing with this approach.

04

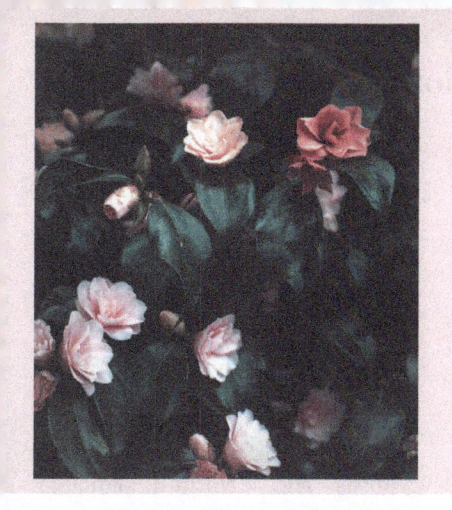

Gut health and rosacea

I carried on digging through the studies, listening to podcasts and reading articles by functional medicine practitioners about rosacea and other skin conditions. The topic that kept coming back was gut abnormalities in relation to all sorts of skin conditions. A relationship between two distinctly different areas was indeed confirmed by many studies- most rosacea sufferers have some kind of gut issue, often without even being aware of it. What is significant, those uncertain gut abnormalities are also linked to all sorts of chronic inflammations. Let me clarify what 'gut issues' I am talking about here and why a healthy gastrointestinal tract plays a crucial role in our overall health.

Gut abnormalities can take place across gut microflora as **gut dysbiosis, SIBO** (small intestine bacteria overgrowth) or can apply to the gut lining that is not working properly and becomes preamble **(leaky gut syndrome)**. Simply speaking, if you have rosacea, it is worth taking all of these gut conditions into account and learning about available tests and treatments.

Gut dysbiosis

Gut dysbiosis is the imbalance between helpful and harmful bacteria (too few healthy 'friendly' bacteria and too many 'unfriendly' ones) in our guts which affects our health negatively.

Advanced gut microbiota studies have revealed a connection between gut dysbiosis and chronic systemic inflammation. However, it remains unclear whether gut dysbiosis is a cause or consequence of the occurring inflammation. What I find very significant is that researchers indicate similar causes for microbiota disruption and chronic systemic inflammation, which are results of a poor diet and lifestyle, stress and use of antibiotics.

> Gut microbiota is the term that stands for the variety of microorganisms living in our gastrointestinal tract, mostly in the intestines (bowels). Gut microorganisms contain communities of bacteria, fungi, viruses and parasites, although bacteria are the most studied. Scientists estimate that there are around 100 trillion microbes living in our gut. Recent years of intense studies have shown that gut microbiome plays a very important role in our health, and although the significance is still being investigated, we already know it's extremely important to our immune system, nervous system, digestion, heart, weight and many other aspects of our health. Some species of microorganism living in our bodies are helpful (beneficial for our health), some are harmful, and some become harmful when we have too much of them.

Studies have also shown that the supplementing of probiotics, particularly species of Lactobacillus, Bifidobacterium, and even Bacillus Coagulans can reduce inflammation.

Leaky Gut

Our gut is covered with special lining that acts as a barrier against the bloodstream. This lining prevents potentially harmful substances from entering our bodies. **But sometimes due to various reasons, the lining becomes permeable** potentially allowing harmful substances like bacteria, toxins, and undigested food particles to enter our bloodstream.

Functional medicine practitioners claim that leaky gut triggers widespread inflammation and stimulates an immune reaction, causing various health problems that are collectively known as leaky gut syndrome. According to many experts, leaky gut can result in autoimmune diseases, migraines, autism, food sensitivities, skin conditions like rosacea, eczema, psoriasis, brain fog, chronic fatigue and many more.

Researchers are not 100% sure what causes leaky gut, but most of them indicate a high level of gluten consumption and bad bacteria overgrowth, a high level of inflammatory mediators and the long-term use of nonsteroidal anti-inflammatory drugs, such as aspirin and ibuprofen, as well as excessive alcohol consumption.

The tests available for leaky gut syndrome reveal the level of zonulin (a protein which controls the size of the openings between your gut lining and your bloodstream) in our systems. Zonulin levels give a good idea of our gut permeability.

It is noticed that people who suffer from rosacea have an

elevated level of zonulin, which indicates leaky gut.

Many experts believe that the integrity of the gut lining is tied to food sensitivities, inflammatory status, liver function, even neurological abnormalities and most probably it affects whole-body health.

SIBO

SIBO stands for Small Intestinal Bacterial Overgrowth which occurs when there is an abnormal increase in the overall bacterial population in the small intestine — particularly bacteria that are not commonly found in that part of the digestive tract.

A study investigated SIBO in rosacea patients and revealed they have a significantly higher SIBO prevalence (60% of rosacea sufferers can be affected by SIBO) than people without this skin condition. That's why antibiotics can often initially work for rosacea by killing the harmful bacteria in the small intestine, but if it is not accompanied by dietary and lifestyle changes and herbal antimicrobial supplementation, SIBO will most probably come back... followed by rosacea.

In my personal opinion, SIBO may be responsible for the vast majority of rosacea cases. I even suspect that I was suffering from SIBO as well because my rosacea was accompanied by various digestive symptoms such as stomach discomfort and belching (typical for this condition) but I believe I managed to suppress it with a low-carb diet, using anti-inflammatory spices such as oregano, as well as intermediate fasting.

Today, I believe it's worth it for any rosacea sufferer to test for SIBO - it is a common root cause of their skin condition. SIBO is relatively easy to treat with medication, herbal therapy and diet but has a tendency to come back. If you test positive for SIBO I recommend you consult your results with a gut specialist, FM practitioner or naturopath to receive guidance and support in overcoming this condition for good.

Testing gut health

These days we can observe a rising awareness in the importance of a balanced gut microbiome for our optimal health. An increasing number of laboratories and companies offer highly advanced tests for gut dysbiosis, leaky gut, gut inflammation and SIBO.

Three years ago, I decided to undertake a stool test for **microbiome dysbiosis and leaky gut which provided a report of my personal microbiome diversity and the condition of my bowels.** A test like that can indicate whether a person's gut bacteria is balanced or if there is a disproportion of some particular microbiome, if there's any inflammation in the gut, or if you have a leaky gut. My test was followed by a free consultation where a professional nutritionist gave me recommendations regarding diet, lifestyle and supplements, all based on my personal results. In my case, the test had shown significant gut dysbiosis plus a leaky gut.

Unfortunately, those tests are not refundable in the UK or in most countries. At the moment, we can only take them privately at a high cost (around £400). Of course, it is everyone's personal preference whether to take a test or not, but I believe it can be the best investment for your own rosacea healing journey, which can finally solve the question: why do I have rosacea? The results can also provide a light on which probiotic would be most suitable for us and on what we need to focus on in regards to our diet.

05

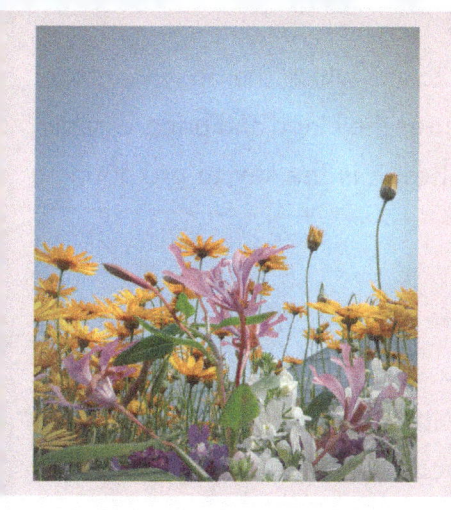

Liver health and rosacea

When I was exploring potential causes of rosacea I noticed that many experts indicate liver congestion as one of the reasons for the development of chronic skin conditions.

Our liver is our body's primary filtration system. It converts toxins into waste products, cleanses our blood, metabolises a wide range of compounds (from nutrients to alcohol and medications), and produces proteins and bile. A healthy liver naturally cleanses itself but if we are exposed to too many harmful substances, over time, our liver can become congested, which means its optimal functioning can be disrupted. If the liver is too congested to filter out all the toxins, our skin will show it through all sorts of conditions and rosacea is believed to be among them.

It is significant that our liver function can be impacted by gut health issues. Our gastrointestinal tracts make an active barrier that helps our bodies to digest and absorb nutrients (into the bloodstream), while at the same time protecting us from unwanted compounds and removing them. If our gut lining is permeable (leaky gut syndrome), toxins which the body wants to get rid of, have the potential to enter the blood and unnecessarily tax the liver. Supporting our gut health is the key to promoting a healthy liver.

Another factor that can cause liver congestion or even damage is chronic stress. When we are stressed or are very anxious, blood flow to the liver is reduced and without adequate blood flow, the liver cannot filter toxins and processed nutrients. Stress also causes inflammation in the liver.

The symptoms that may indicate liver congestion are:

-lack of appetite
-dark urine
-disrupted sleep pattern or exhaustion
-various skin conditions, e.g. rosacea
-foggy memory
-chronic fatigue
-hormone imbalances
-moodiness, anxiousness or depression
-excessive sweating
-inability to lose weight
-unusually pale stools

You can test your liver health by taking an advanced liver-functioning blood test. If you think you will need support and guidance in improving your liver health, I strongly encourage you to speak to your doctor, or to a holistic health practitioner such as a naturopath, nutritionist or functional medicine doctor.

How can we support liver health? The most important thing we can do to have a healthy, well functioning liver is to look after our diet and lifestyle.

Some simple ways to prevent liver congestion are:

- Avoiding alcohol, which is taxing on the liver
- Supporting the liver with a healthy diet
- Avoiding coffee, sodas, and other caffeinated foods and beverages
- Avoiding sugar
- Avoiding toxins and pesticides in foods by consuming organic products
- Avoiding environmental toxins as much as possible
- Exercising regularly to increase blood flow to the liver
- Drinking plenty of water every day
- Managing your stress on a daily basis
- Keeping your other organs in good overall health

For more information on how to improve your liver health with your diet go to <u>Liver friendly diet</u> subchapter (p.51).

To end this chapter, I would like to highlight that we cannot cleanse or boost liver health overnight. It takes time to improve the liver function, a minimum of a couple of months is needed and in order to do it, you need to look holistically at your overall wellbeing, including mental health.

These days, more than ever before, we are constantly exposed to environmental toxins, pollution, chemicals in our everyday cosmetics and household products, plastic, preservatives, and other artificial substances in our food. All these factors over time cause an accumulation of harmful compounds in the body and can cause a burden on our livers, as well as the rest of our body's complex detoxification pathways and organs (skin, gut, lungs, spleen, lymphatic system, kidneys).

If you suffer from rosacea it is crucial for you to avoid whenever possible these harmful substances, by choosing organic unprocessed foods, natural cosmetics, house cleaning products, etc. It might also be a good idea to consider detoxing daily as part of a proactive rosacea healing journey.

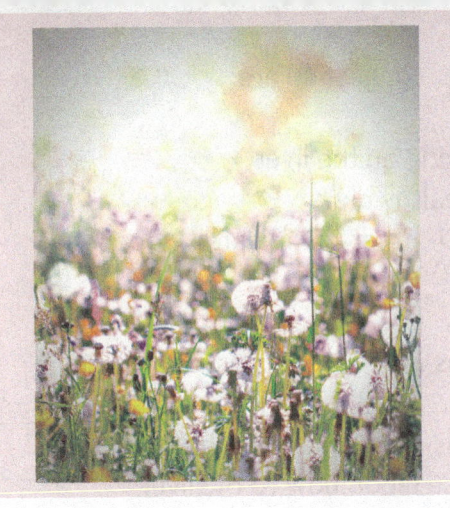

06

Do Demodex mites cause rosacea?

Demodex mites are microorganisms which naturally live within the human body, especially on our skin - they are part of our microbiome.

There has been much debate as to whether their increased numbers are a cause or result of rosacea. However, evidence appears to be mounting up that an overabundance of Demodex mites may possibly trigger an immune response in people with rosacea, or that the inflammation may be caused by certain bacteria associated with the mites. The medical world has noticed that the mites are most plentiful in the same regions of the face that are most commonly affected by rosacea - the cheeks, nose, chin and forehead - and that large quantities of mites have been found in biopsies of rosacea papules and pustules.

According to Dr Martin Schaller, assistant professor of dermatology at Ludwig-Maximilians University in Munich, Germany, severe infestation of Demodex mites, known as demodicosis, **rather mimics the symptoms of rosacea but it is not actually rosacea.**

On the other hand, functional medicine practitioners indicate that if the body itself is imbalanced and there's a microbiome dysbiosis in the gut, the skin microbiome will be interrupted as well and the population of Demodex mites can grow.

In my opinion, it is always worth trying topical medication against mites (like Soolantra cream- you will need a prescription for this one) with rosacea symptoms and see how your skin responds to it. If within a couple of weeks, you see no improvement, it means the root causes for your rosacea lay much deeper. It may also be the case that you will see a limited improvement and once again, this indicates that internal body healing is needed to reverse your rosacea.

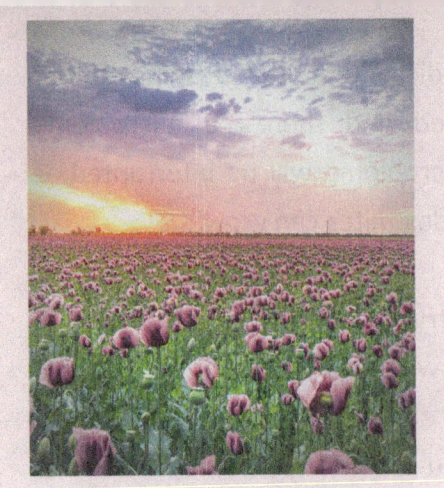

07

Time to reflect- what caused my rosacea

My knowledge and awareness of the connection between rosacea, chronic inflammation and gut/liver abnormalities were growing gradually and thanks to functional medicine, everything started to make sense. At some point, I felt ready to put into practice everything I had learnt so far in order to tackle my skin inflammation. The first step was to reflect critically on my general health, on my diet and lifestyle. For way too long I had been avoiding this moment, thinking to myself that life is unfair as I was eating much healthier than others and they didn't have rosacea, yet I did.

But now I was ready to stop comparing myself, to stop ruminating over my bad skin and to finally take a critical look at my own habits in order to understand what I needed to do to heal my skin. I must say, the process of reflecting upon your lifestyle in a fault-finding way is emotionally difficult and intimidating, but it is inevitable if you want to heal any chronic skin condition. **As functional medicine finds, all chronic skin conditions are the manifestation of something awry inside the** body; to heal any skin condition, you must eliminate the cause for it.

To be fair, we are very lucky because these days, there are many extensive studies on chronic conditions and gut and liver abnormalities that indicate the most probable grounds for our problems. Now all we need to do is to use the reference points to check ourselves. Being brutally honest and thorough in our self-reflection is crucial.

Today, over three years after I changed my habits to gain clear skin, reflecting back at my pre-rosacea lifestyle isn't that hard for me anymore as I now have a full perspective. I am not surprised that I had rosacea. For way too long, I didn't bother thinking about what was good or bad for my body or mind, and to be fair, I didn't really appreciate my health that much; I took it for granted. Of course, I wanted to be healthy but I had always believed it was due to luck and when people developed chronic conditions, it was a misfortune. Today, my view on this matter has turned 180 degrees. Obviously, no one chooses to be poorly, no one wants to suffer, and no one even wishes to deal with skin issues. We don't plan it, we definitely don't intend for it, but it doesn't mean that we don't do it to ourselves. Sadly, most people don't have awareness on how the modern diet and lifestyle affects their health. Most people don't even have time to stop and think about it or conduct any research on this topic.

Thanks to rosacea, I found motivation and willingness to dedicate my time to my own health. I wanted to go through a reflective journey to understand my wrongs and to find a new, healthier way of living that would serve my wellbeing.

Below I list the causes which I believe triggered my skin inflammation. However I am unable to determine which one started my rosacea symptoms. Intuitively, I feel like it wasn't one particular reason; I think it was more of a combination and an accumulation of various poor dietary, health and lifestyle habits.

> I would like to encourage you to take some paper and a pencil while you are reading my pro-inflammatory habits confession, and reflect on your own life. Can you see any similarities in your own habits?

Poor diet. My diet was never 'terrible' (I know people who ate much worse than I used to) because I always ate at least the recommended five portions of fruit and vegetables a day. But on top of that, I would eat lots of processed foods (deli meats, salty snacks, sweets, take-aways at least once a week), loads of carbohydrates and gluten (pasta, bread and plain flour used to be a base for nearly all my meals), and deep-fried foods. I also wasn't paying enough attention to the ingredient lists on the products I was regularly buying and consuming. I would consume lots of foods like processed meats and pâtés which I used to love, and others that contained preservatives, artificial flavour enrichments and stabilisers. Furthermore, I would often overeat or eat my meals in a rush. I would also snack a lot, and I wasn't ever giving my digestive system a chance to rest and regenerate.

Unhealthy, irregular sleep patterns. I have always been a light sleeper. My rosacea first appeared when my little boy was around ten months old. He was waking up regularly throughout the night, so I didn't sleep properly for months. A lack of good rest and chronic exhaustion not only makes us feel demotivated and irritable, but also contributes to microbe dysbiosis in our guts - one of the factors linked to chronic inflammation.

Too much stress and anxiety. When we stress, our bodies release stress hormones into our systems. Over time, this can contribute to microbe dysbiosis and body inflammation and can affect liver functions.

I have always been an easily stressed person. That came from my upbringing. There was always lots of tension, arguments, pressure and a nervous atmosphere around me when I was growing up. Mostly, we learn and absorb all these negative patterns unconsciously when we are children. In my adult life, chronic stress used to affect all aspects of my existence – my physical health, mental state, emotional stability and relationships with people.

In the past, I used to cultivate stress. I believed stressing was caring. I cared and wanted to control everything. I was always worrying, rushing, putting lots of pressure on myself and surrounded myself with lots of negativity. Back then, I also didn't appreciate any 'me time', the need for daily relaxation and unwinding after (and/or before) a busy and hectic day. I didn't allow myself any time for mental hygiene. I felt overwhelmed and stressed out every day.

Too little physical activity. Working out was always very low on my list of priorities and since I had small kids, I could always find more important things to do rather than any physical exercise. What I wasn't aware of was that when we move our muscles, our bodies release anti-inflammatory molecules into our systems. Sedentary lifestyles contribute to poor health and inflammation.

Relying on antibiotics and over-the-counter medications. One year before rosacea started to appear on my face, I kept having frequent ear infections and also mastitis during breastfeeding (a milk canal infection). I took around eight courses of antibiotics within a one-year period (and I didn't supplement with any probiotics as nobody mentioned them to me at that time). On top of that, I was regularly taking painkillers like paracetamol or ibuprofen for headaches, period cramps and colds. Unfortunately, antibiotics cause havoc to good bacteria in our guts, and all the medications contribute to gut lining permeability and load on our liver.

I was overwhelming my skin with tonnes of skincare and make-up products which were filled with harmful chemicals. I was into commercial pictures of beauty and health and I believed that I just had to use loads of various cosmetics to achieve good-looking skin or I had to use expensive perfumes to smell beautifully all day. On top of that I was using harsh household cleaning products because I only looked at what was effective rather then the toxicity of it. Constant exposure to harmful substances puts an extra load on the liver and has a negative effect on its optimal functioning.

08

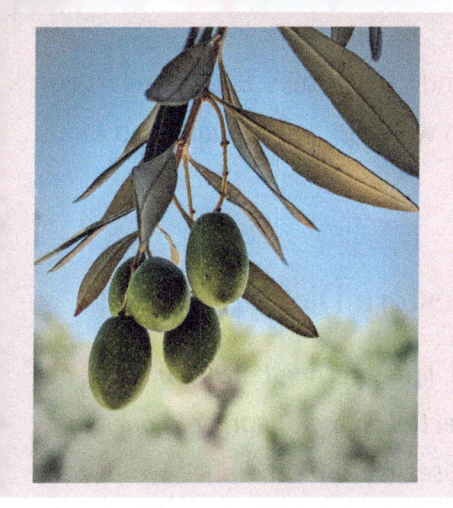

Rosacea healing diets

This chapter I consider to be the most important part of this book. Why? Because according to many experts, the right nutrition plays the key role in reversing rosacea and preventing it from coming back. My own experience with rosacea confirms this presumption. In this chapter I'm going to pass on to you the most important information on how your diet relates to rosacea and your optimal health, but also how you can use the food as a medicine that treats and prevents skin inflammation.

I am also going to present you with all the practical changes I have made in terms of my diet that enabled me to heal my own skin. I will talk about building new awareness when it comes to nutrition and new (but now continuing) dietary habits that helped me to reverse rosacea for good.

All the information included in this chapter is based on my own research, personal consultations with holistic health professionals (like nutritionists and naturopaths), and finally my own experience.

Again, I would encourage you to explore further all the topics discussed in this chapter (and beyond!). Expanding your awareness in health and nutrition will help you to make conscious and effective lifestyle shifts.

Modern Western Diet

"For most people across the world, life is getting better but diets are getting worse. This is the bittersweet dilemma of eating in our times. Unhealthy food, eaten in a hurry, seems to be the price we pay for living in liberated modern societies."- Bee Wilson in The Guardian.

When I started learning about body inflammation and I came across the fact that, according to all the most recent research, modern Western diet plays an important role in destabilising our gut microbes, causing leaky gut, overwhelming our liver, causing chronic inflammation in our bodies and being responsible for widespread chronic autoimmunological conditions.

Therefore modern diet is where our discussion must begin. We already know that our typical western diet is composed of way too much sugar, starch, gluten, salt, alcohol, caffeine and deep-fried food (including takeaways). There are too few wholefoods, plants, healthy Omega 3 fats, herbs, vitamins and minerals, and not enough fibre and antioxidants. Now, I would like us to look deeper into this topic and explore why the main elements of modern diet are so bad for our health.

Too much carbohydrates in our diet.
Carbohydrates are basically what modern diets are based on. They can be vegan, vegetarian, pescatarian or classic

diets which include meat. Sugar, bread, pastries, grains, potatoes, alcohol, snacks etc. - we consume carbs all the time. Yes, carbs make a source of energy for humans but at the same time, they feed all the pathogens (did you know that microbes, with a few very rare exceptions, can only survive if fed with carbs?). Excessive gluten consumption (which is a component of grains like wheat, spelt, and rye) is also being recognised as a factor that causes gut lining permeability, allowing toxins that should exit, to circulate in our systems and causing all sorts of modern chronic conditions.

Studies also confirm that eating too many carbs can negatively affect our ability to control blood sugar levels (people who eat a carb-rich diet face a higher risk of developing type-2 diabetes).

Mass produced foods are very low quality.
These poor-quality foods start from farming. Mass production farming uses a wide range of chemicals (e.g. pesticides) to protect plants from insects, to make them bigger and more resilient. Livestock is given antibiotics, growth hormones and is fed low-quality fodder (mostly the cheapest grains, not their natural foods). This affects their welfare and completely changes the nutritional aspects of the meat, dairy and eggs, often making them more harmful than beneficial for humans.

Foods are highly processed and contain artificial additives.
Further along this path, mass food producers know that modern consumers like to have 'very easy life' when it comes to food preparation. Spending only a little time in the kitchen but having ready meals available on demand is preferred. Food producers know their demands, what the consumers don't often realise is

that the easy, convenient food, packed snacks, sweets and processed foods are very often filled with artificial additives such as monosodium glutamate, propylene glycol or sodium nitrite to name a few. This makes them last longer (cost-effectiveness for producers) and look and taste better (to ensure customer demand).

We also often don't even realise that those artificial substances are in fact toxic chemicals, which have a very negative effect on our health if consumed regularly. "Hang on a minute" - you must think - surely, there are some tests, regulations and controls on which food additives are safe to use and which are not, and food producers can not put poison in our foods? Yes, there are regulations but all tests are carried out in a short period of time on a very moderate amount of these substances. Small amounts of synthetic additives won't kill us right away. But what about if we consume them for years regularly? How to test it? Who would volunteer to apply a toxin to their system for a long time?

Let's look at sodium nitrite. A preservative commonly added to deli meats, bacon, sausages, gammon, etc. The lab tests on rats (and there were so many of those tests) showed that even very small amounts taken regularly can cause liver cancer. Nitrites are banned from use in foods in Norway and Sweden but are still commonly used in the UK, USA, Europe and other countries. In fact, you can challenge yourself - go to the biggest supermarket in your town and try to find a ham or bacon without sodium nitrate...

Too little Omega3 /too much Omega6.

While both Omega fats (3 and 6) are important for our body functions, getting their balance right is where the problem begins. In modern societies, we don't eat enough Omega3 fats found in foods like sea fish, seafood, walnuts, flaxseeds, chia seeds and organic pasture-raised animal products. Instead, we consume way too much Omega6 which is commonly found in the refined oils and foods cooked in them, as well as in mass-farmed animal products. Omega3 fats have anti-inflammatory properties whereas too much Omega6 in our diet increases the risk of chronic inflammation and inflammatory diseases.

Not enough fibre and antioxidants.

In a modern Western diet, we eat too little fibre which feeds our gut bacteria and has a 'cleansing' effect on our digestive tract. Our food also lacks antioxidants which protect our cells from free radicals damage and keep inflammation in check.

Eating in a rush, constant snacking and eating too big quantities.
These negative eating habits simply overwhelm our digestive systems. When we're consuming our food in a rush, we don't chew it properly. This means we skip the first important step in digesting food- breaking it down by saliva enzymes. The purpose of these enzymes is to start digesting and lubricating what we eat. Without chewing food for long enough, our digestive tract has to work harder to break down foods that should already be partially processed. Constant snacking doesn't allow our digestive tract to ever rest and regenerate. It is not natural for humans to eat all the time and it causes our digestive system to be in a constant state of alert.

Last but not least, modern societies eat too much food (and sadly poor quality), expecting their digestive systems to break down the quantities that they are not adjusted to deal with.

Relying on supplements for nutrient intake.
Getting nutrients, vitamins, minerals and antioxidants into our bodies is obviously good. However, doing it through supplements may not make any difference to our health and in some cases can be more harmful than beneficial. How come?

Firstly, nutrients don't work well without the presence of other nutrients, which we get more naturally through a well-balanced diet.

Secondly, the supplements you take may interact with each other (if you're taking more than one) as well as with medications you may be taking.

Lastly, we forget that supplements are also heavily processed products. In order to give them a long-shelf life and keep the desired consistency and shape, they often contain synthetic substances (such as binders, fillers, glazing agents, preservatives).

Anti-inflammatory diet as an opposition to a modern diet

These days we hear about so many people suffering from various chronic inflammatory conditions: rosacea, eczema, psoriasis, Hashimoto's, Crohn's, etc. to name a few. They affect Western populations more and more every year. At the same time, extensive studies continue to deliver more precise data on diet and lifestyle in relation to chronic inflammation. There is so much evidence at this point that our diets act as catalysts for chronic inflammation or as defenders that protect us from it.

We already know that the modern Western diet is the one to blame for the widespread of modern autoimmunological conditions. So what is the alternative?

Anti-inflammatory diet

It is an eating pattern that is thought to reduce, heal and prevent all sorts of chronic body inflammation and associated diseases and maintain general health and vitality. The foundation for this diet is a belief that what you eat can play either a positive or negative role in managing chronic inflammation.

Fundamentally this diet is focused on whole foods – vegetables, fruits (low in sugar fruits like berries), organic pasture-raised meat and eggs, nuts, sea fish and other sources of healthy fats and minimal grains consumption. An anti-inflammatory diet rejects highly processed foods with artificial additives, foods high in sugars, excessive amounts of grains, starch and dairy as they all affect our gut. Instead, it supports gut health and good microbe variety with various, colourful meals full of fibre, and antioxidants.

The anti-inflammatory diet is often associated with the Mediterranean diet which also focuses on freshly cooked food, a big variety of vegetables rich in antioxidants, healthy Omega3 fats (from fish, seafood, olive oil, seeds and nuts), high-quality products coming from free-range farming, and natural agriculture. In both Mediterranean and anti-inflammatory diets, the meals are colourful, fresh and appealing.

I personally believe an anti-inflammatory diet is a long-term answer to rosacea as well as other inflammatory conditions. This diet is varied and satisfying. Following its rules doesn't stop us from eating out occasionally (avoiding takeaways though) because we can always find something suitable (e.g. grilled fish and steamed vegetables or salads with simple olive oil dressing).

> There are different variations of anti-inflammatory diets regarding grains. Initially, healthy wholegrains were promoted to be consumed every day. Now with all the recent knowledge about how carbs can affect our gut health, anti-inflammatory tendencies go toward minimizing grain consumption (especially those with gluten); they are still included in this diet but not in large quantities.

After about three months of focusing on my gut health, I moved gradually to eating the anti-inflammatory diet and this is when I noticed that my skin started to heal. What I consider to be my success is that at this point, I didn't make the classic mistake of returning to my old eating habits. Instead, I kept going with an anti-inflammatory diet. I actually started to enjoy eating healthily and appreciated how it made me feel and look. My body became toned and for the first time in my life I received compliments on my glowing complexion!

If you are a rosacea sufferer, I strongly advise you to nurture the topic of anti-inflammatory diets as much as you can and implement it in your life as soon as possible. There are many books available; cookbooks, articles, podcasts, videos, and even magazines dedicated to anti-inflammatory diets, to help us understand what to eat to be healthy.

Anti-inflammatory diet rules:
-avoid too many grains (especially with gluten) and starch in your diet
-avoid sugars and alcohol (only an occasional glass of red wine)
-eat lots of healthy fats
-eat a variety of vegetables, salads and berry fruits
-cook from fresh, organic ingredients
-use lots of anti-inflammatory herbs and spices
-exclude processed foods and takeaways from your diet

Examples of anti-inflammatory meals:

Breakfast

Eggs in all forms, shakshuka, roasted or smoked salmon, or other fish with gluten-free toast.
Porridge with toppings like coconut flakes, 100% cocoa nibs or powder, chia seeds, flaxseeds, berries (fresh or frozen) and avocado.

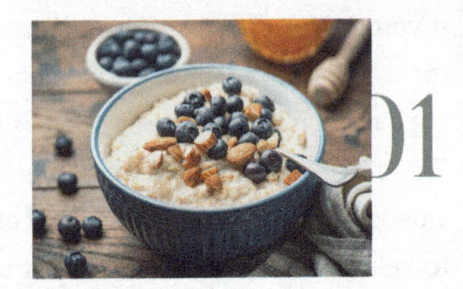

Lunch

Homemade gluten-free pitas with roasted veg, gluten-free sandwiches with eggs and/or salmon, salads (lots of green leaves, tomatoes, olives, red onion, cucumber, broccoli sprouts) with roasted organic meat, wild fish or eggs with a simple dressing of olive oil and lemon/lime juice. Homemade smoothies.

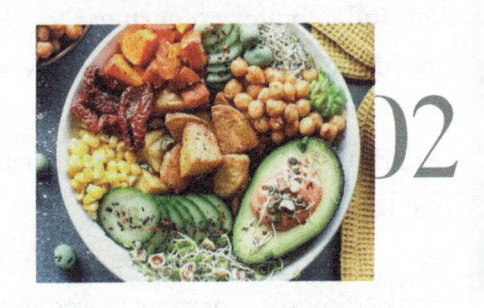

Snack

Berries, a handful of walnuts or almonds; coconut yogurt, an orange. black grapes. Hummus with vegetable sticks. Falafels, a couple of pieces of dark chocolate (min 85% cocoa solids).

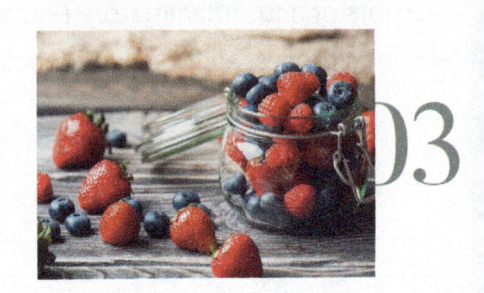

Dinner

Vegetable and meat stews, curries with chicken, beef or fish served with a small amount of millet, quinoa or rice, gluten-free pastas, boiled potatoes or sweet potatoes with a large portion of veg and a piece of meat or fish. Homemade soups, homemade oven chips with lots of herbs like oregano, sage, thyme and dried garlic.

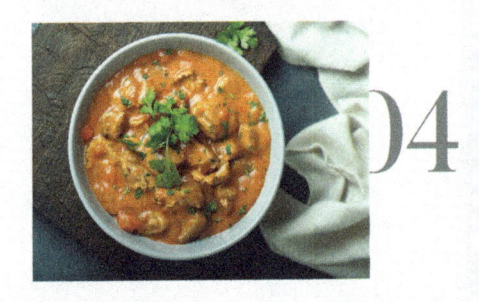

Gut healing diets

Following an anti-inflammatory diet for the long term, in my opinion, is the best option to maintain optimal health (including in the gut and liver), to keep any chronic inflammation in check without compromising on joy and satisfaction from eating. But if your gut health is already disturbed (I believe that gut abnormalities and rosacea are strongly connected), I encourage you to first focus on fixing the existing gut problem and then gradually move towards a more intuitive and diverse anti-inflammatory diet.

Why? Because an anti-inflammatory diet does allow moderate amounts of grains, healthy sugars (from fruits) and starchy vegetables like potatoes. But generally speaking, carbohydrates actively feed and encourage microbes, which can cause inflammation and be detrimental to our gut health.

By contrast, diets based only on fat and fibre are unfriendly to invading microbes. If you have guts dysbiosis, a low-carb diet, supplementing with probiotics and regularly eating fermented foods (my favourite is sauerkraut) can be very helpful by bringing back the optimal balance to your gut microbiome.

If you suffer from a leaky gut, which is very common for rosacea sufferers, you will need your diet to be full of gut-rebuilding substances like gelatine and free amino acids (e.g. proline and glycine). You should also rest your digestive system regularly (see Intermittent fasting subchapter, p.54) to give it a chance to regenerate, heal and rebuild.

If you have SIBO on the other hand (small intestine bacteria overgrowth), you may need a proper treatment with either medications or natural remedies or both. The most effective SIBO treatments should be supported by certain diets, which colloquially speaking, should starve the bacteria in your small intestine. For years a low FODMAP diet was promoted to be successful in 'killing' SIBO but these days many gut specialists point out that this diet still contains lots of sugar, starch and fibre. Yes, fibre is problematic here as well since SIBO doesn't mean there's a 'bad' microbe in your small intestine, it may be 'good' microbe but it is too much of it where it shouldn't be). It also provides lots of food for bacteria, So a low FODMAP diet can not be effective in SIBO treatment. Instead, many professionals recommend a GAPs diet or a Ketogenic diet against SIBO.

These two diets, especially the GAPs diet are a very good solution for all sorts of gut dysfunctions and I highly recommend learning more about it.

> According to GAPs Diet and its founder Dr Natasha Campbell-McBride, the most gut-healing food that we can consume is homemade meat stock (e.g. chicken stock) made of the bones and meat attached to them. What's more, Dr Campbell-McBride claims that meat stock is better than bone broth if the primary focus is on healing the gut. Bone broth is ideal for consuming once gut healing has taken place.
>
> The significant difference is that the meat stock is not cooked as long as bone broth. Meat stock is especially rich in gelatine and free amino acids, like proline and glycine. These amino acids, along with the gelatinous protein from the meat and connective tissue, are particularly beneficial in healing and strengthening connective tissue found in the lining of the gut. These nutrients are pulled out of the meat and connective tissue during the first several hours of cooking meaty fish, poultry, beef and lamb (the larger the bones, the longer the recommended cooking time). The amino acids (except for histidine) are present in higher amounts in bone broth and for people with a leaky gut, the high concentration of some amino acids may be problematic.

low FODMAP diet

This diet is low in fermentable carbs.

A low FODMAP diet restricts certain foods that are high in fermentable sugars (they're not digestible and gut bacteria ferment them, increasing gas and short-chain fatty acid production).

Foods to avoid on a low FODMAP diet:
- wheat, rye, nuts, legumes, artichokes, garlic, and onion
- lactose-containing products such as milk, yogurt, soft cheese, ice cream, buttermilk, condensed milk, and whipped cream
- fructose-containing foods, including fruits such as apples, pears, watermelon, and mango and sweeteners such as honey, agave nectar, and high fructose corn syrup
- mannitol and sorbitol in apples, stone fruits, cauliflower, mushrooms, and snow peas, as well as xylitol and isomalt in low-calorie sweeteners, such as those in sugar-free gum and mints

This diet is often recommended to manage irritable bowel syndrome (IBS);

Ketogenic diet

This term stands for a low-carb diet (like the Atkins diet). The idea is to get more calories from protein and fat and less from carbohydrates.

Foods that are generally allowed include high-fat meats, fish, oils, nuts, high-fat dairy such as cheese, and low-carb vegetables such as leafy greens.

Reducing carb levels means cutting out bread, pasta, rice, and baked goods, but also legumes, root vegetables, most fruits and starchy veggies, such as potatoes.

GAPs diet

This diet was invented by Dr Natasha Campbell-McBride, who believes that poor nutrition and a leaky gut, or increased intestinal permeability, are responsible for many psychological, neurological, behavioural issues and auto-immunological conditions.

Dr Campbell-McBride's initial aim with the GAPS diet was to help children with behavioural disorders. However, with the newest studies on gut permeability and gut microbiome, it has become clear that disturbed gut health can result with all sorts of chronic conditions, so common in modern societies.

At the core of the GAPS diet, is to heal the gut by avoiding foods that are difficult to digest and might damage the gut flora or gut lining such as grains, commercial dairy, starchy foods and all processed and refined carbohydrates;

Instead, GAPs diet promotes eating nutrient-rich foods that help the gut to heal, such as organic meat broth and fermented food, organic meat and eggs, wild fish, organic vegetables.

Please note that people with disturbed gut health often have many food sensitivities (intolerances) and can be also sensitive to histamine-rich foods (like tomatoes, avocados, hard cheeses, etc). While healing your gut, you should exclude all the foods you are aware to be intolerant to (or you believe you are) as they can irritate your bowel and increase inflammation. After a period of working on your gut health, you can slowly start reintroducing previously intolerant foods and observe how your body reacts.

I drew my inspiration and knowledge about gut healing foods from the GAPs diet and even though I wasn't very strict with its guidelines, I included their critical steps during my gut healing stage:

- no gluten at all
- eating only cooked vegetables (easier to digest), meat and eggs (organic if possible), sea fish and seafood
- consuming homemade meat stock (almost) every day
- no dairy, sugar or alcohol
- no processed foods and no takeaways
- consuming homemade fermented foods
- intermittent fasting

Ways to support your gut health

1. Testing your gut health

2. Supplementing with probiotics

3. Increasing fibre in your diet

4. Drinking homemade chicken broth

5. Avoiding antibiotics and over the counter medications

6. Eating fermented foods (not on low-histamine diet)

Gut Healing Organic Chicken Stock

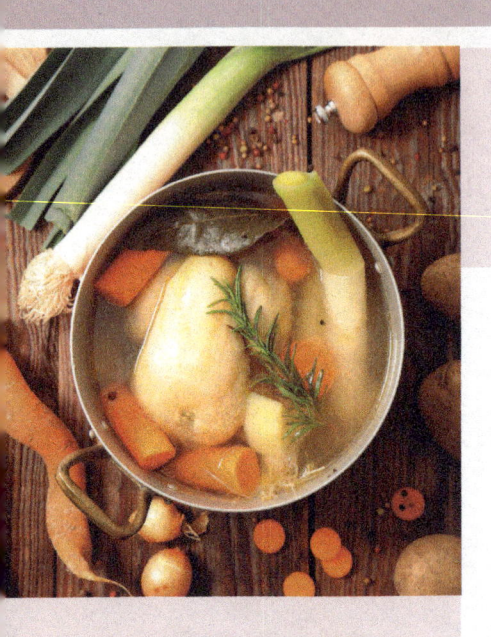

PREP TIME: LESS THAN 10 MIN

COOKING TIME APPROX. 2 HOURS

INGREDIENTS

1 whole organic chicken
2-4 organic chicken feet (optional- for extra gelatine)
4 or more litres of filtered water
1-2 medium yellow onions
2-4 carrots
2-4 celery sticks or 1/4 of celeriac root
3-5 garlic cloves
a couple of bay leaves
1 tablespoon of raw apple cider vinegar (optional- to get more of the minerals and trace elements out of the bones)
1-3 teaspoons of mineral salt
bunch of parsley

DIRECTION

- Rinse the chicken in clean fresh water.
- Place it in the pan and add the remaining ingredients.
- Fill the pan with filtered water.
- Bring to a boil. Reduce the heat to a simmer and cook for 1 ½ to 2 hours.
- Add parsley and salt during the last 10 minutes of cooking.

NOTES

When the chicken soup is ready, you can debone the chicken and reserve it for eating or putting it back into the stock.

You can eat the chicken stock as a soup in a bowl with added chicken meat and carrots or drink the stock from a cup (use a fine sieve to pour it into the cup if you don't want any little bits, just a clear stock).

Liver-friendly diet

We have already discussed that liver congestion and dysfunctions can contribute to rosacea. Fortunately, we can improve our liver's function by supporting it on a regular basis. Some people decide to go on a liver cleanse, which usually means drinking lots of fresh vegetable juices. A liver cleanse usually lasts up to a couple of weeks and it's an intentional reset of the liver's natural detoxifying functions.

In my opinion, doing a radical detox but then going back to liver overwhelming diet and lifestyle, can only bring short-term fixes.

For many rosacea sufferers, improving their liver health will instead require permanent dietary and lifestyle changes. Personally, I am a fan of natural means of supporting the liver through diet and natural supplements, so it can perform optimally and detoxify naturally. However, if you decide to go on a liver detox program I encourage you to do it under the supervision of a licensed functional medicine practitioner, naturopath or nutritionist.

The main strategy to keep your liver healthy is to adopt a liver-friendly diet.

First of all, eating a balanced, plant-dense diet that contains diverse nutrients and phytonutrients is what supports liver and gut health. Focusing on whole foods (organic when possible)- including vegetables, fruits, beans, nuts, seeds, free-range organic meats and eggs, wild fish, healthy grains and minimally processed oils, such as olive, avocado, or coconut oil.

Avoiding all processed foods, convenient foods and anything with artificial additives, as well as takeaways, deep-fried foods and refined oils.

Drinking lots of water: 8-10 glasses of filtered water every day. Drinking warm water (with optional freshly squeezed lemon juice) is best as it helps digestion and optimal functioning of the lymphatic system, which both support liver health and the body's detoxification pathways.

Looking after your gut health - supporting optimal gut barrier function will help to reduce the number of toxins that enter your bloodstream (which your liver has to filter and remove). Minimalizing gluten consumption and eating regularly meat stock can help to rebuild your gut lining. Adding to your diet fermenting foods loaded with probiotic bacteria that promote healthy digestion and the integrity of the gut lining, will help to keep toxins out of the bloodstream.

Avoiding alcohol- excessive alcohol consumption is one of the leading causes of liver damage.

Adding to your diet foods that promote healthy liver functioning (foods which fuel glutathione production, bind heavy metals/toxins and help stimulate bile flow) such as almonds, salmon, avocado, artichokes, berries, broccoli sprouts, beetroots, cruciferous vegetables (such as broccoli, cabbage, cauliflower, brussels sprouts), watercress and dark leafy greens, lentils, green tea, citrus fruits; also natural supplements like chlorella, dandelion root, milk thistle, turmeric and vitamin C.

Not overeating and looking after your body weight. It is proven that high levels of body fat have a negative impact on liver health.

Practising intermittent fasting which promotes additional liver detox support.

Intermittent fasting

Have you ever heard of intermittent fasting? Before my rosacea healing journey, I only heard about it from a friend as an effective method to lose weight, but I wasn't ever attracted to this idea. When I started educating myself about rosacea, chronic body inflammations and gut and liver health, I noticed that many experts advise intermittent fasting as a way for natural detoxing and cell repair.

Intermittent fasting is the daily 16-hour fast, in which you limit all of your daily eating to an 8-hour window and fast for the remaining 16 hours. Let's say the last meal was consumed at 6 pm, then your next meal would be around 10 the following morning.

"Periods without food give our body [including gut and liver] a chance to repair and clean itself out since it doesn't have to focus on or funnel energy to our digestive system"- William Cole, D.C, functional medicine expert.

Clinical research shows that intermittent fasting has numerous health benefits like reducing insulin resistance, improving various metabolic features that are important for brain health. It also reduces the risk of cancer. But what really should interest rosacea sufferers is that fasting induces the cellular repair processes, and triggers a metabolic pathway (called autophagy), which removes waste material from cells and reduces inflammation in the body.

Conscious grocery shopping

Since I am now aware of how processed foods can impact our health, I believe it is very important to read the ingredient lists on all the products we buy and eliminate everything from our trollies that has any artificial additives. You can learn the names of additives to avoid (preservatives, glutamines, stabilisers, etc.) but ultimately, I would avoid any ingredients sounding 'strange'. Instead, I would only buy products made of good, natural components I know and recognise.

Obviously, I encourage you to cook as much as you can from scratch but sometimes buying something processed is unavoidable. For example, I allow my kids to have store-bought snacks but I always make sure I buy the best possible options with regard to flavour and health benefits. Going on an anti-inflammatory diet has definitely turned me into a conscious buyer and consumer. Initially, when I made the shift towards conscious living, I had to substitute lots of products and brands that I used to buy (products like ketchup, mayo, sausages, etc.) with ones including simple ingredients. It was quite tricky at the beginning to introduce my family to slightly different flavours but now they prefer the healthy options– our taste preferences change in line with what we consume regularly.

You should always stay vigilant during shopping because even foods that you would never expect to contain synthetic additives are culprits of unnecessary tampering (for example olives or breads). Also, foods marked as organic or natural can contain harmful additives, therefore I encourage you to always check the ingredients label on the back of the packaging.

At the same time, I must reassure you that there are currently so many fantastic brands that sell natural and 'nasty additives'-free products, so you don't need to worry that you will starve on a healthy diet. My family and I certainly don't!

I have mentioned many times in this chapter that gluten is bad for our gut and regular gluten consumption can contribute to rosacea. Yet, I would like to warn you - 'gluten-free' labelled products: gluten-free breads, flatbreads, biscuits, pasta, etc. often contain tonnes of artificial additives. I encourage you to be cautious, read those labels and only choose the products with clean and simple compositions.

Here are examples of the ingredient lists within the same types of products; I put ✓ by the ones I would choose and ✗ by the ones I wouldn't buy due to bad composition.

ALMOND MILK
Ingredients lists from four different brands

| Water, Almond (2.3%), Calcium [Tri-Calcium Phosphate], Sea Salt, **Stabilisers (Locust Bean Gum, Gellan Gum), Emulsifier (Lecithins (Sunflower))**, Vitamins (B2, B12, E, D2) ✗ | Water, Almonds (2%), Calcium, **Acidity Regulator:E340, Stabiliser:E418, E417, Sunflower Lecithin**, Sea Salt, Potassium Iodide, Vitamin B12, Vitamin D ✗ | Spring Water, Almonds (4.5%), Seaweed Lithothamnium Calcareum* and Sea Salt

*Seaweed as a natural source of Calcium ✓ | Spring Water, Rice, Italian Almonds (1%), Sunflower Oil, Calcium Carbonate, Sea Salt ✓ |

SAUSAGES For My Family
Ingredients lists from five different brands

Outdoor Bred Pork (90%), Water, Gluten Free Crumb (Rice Flour, Chickpea Flour, Cornflour, Salt, Dextrose), Sea Salt, Ground Spices (White Pepper, Coriander, Nutmeg), Dried Onion, **Stabiliser: E450, Preservative: E223 (Sulphites),** Antioxidant: Ascorbic Acid, Sausages filled into Natural Pork Casings	Pork (90%), Water, Potato Starch, Salt, Dextrose, Spices (Pepper, Nutmeg), Herbs (Sage, Parsley), **Stabiliser (Triphosphates), Preservative (Sodium Sulphite),** Antioxidant (Ascorbic Acid), Spice Extracts, Acidity Regulator (Citric Acid), Sage Extract, Filled into Natural Pork Casings D	British or Irish Pork (90%), Water, Sea Salt, Flavouring, Rice Flour, Chickpea Flour, Ground Spices (Coriander, White Pepper, Nutmeg), Dried Onion, Antioxidant: Ascorbic Acid, Salt, Cornflour, Dextrose, Sausages filled into Natural Vegetable Casings	Organic British Pork (95%), Sea Salt*, Breadcrumbs (Fortified Wheat Flour (Wheat Flour, Calcium Carbonate*, Iron*, Niacin*, Thiamin*), Salt*, Yeast*), Water*, Onion Powder, Rusk (Fortified Wheat Flour (Wheat Flour, Calcium Carbonate*, Iron*, Niacin*, Thiamin*), Yeast*, Salt*), Sage, Coriander, Nutmeg, White Pepper, Antioxidant: Ascorbic Acid*.	
✗	✗	✓	✓	

OLIVES
Ingredients lists from three different brands

Black Olives (91%) [Pitted Black Olives, Salt, **Stabiliser (Ferrous Gluconate)**], Sunflower Oil	Hojiblanca Olives, Water, Pimento (1.9 %), Salt, **Thickener (Sodium Alginate, Guar Gum)**, Acidity Regulator (Citric Acid)	Nocellara Olives (94%) (Green Olives, Salt), Sunflower Oil
✗	✗	✓

GLUTEN-FREE BREAD
Ingredients lists from four different brands

Gluten Free Flour (Tapioca Starch, Potato Starch, Rice Flour, Cornflour), Sunflower Oil, Water, Millet Flakes (3%), Bamboo Fibre, **Stabiliser: E464, E466, Xanthan Gum,** Dried Egg White, Sugar, **Humectant: Glycerol**, Yeast (Yeast, Vitamin D Yeast), Psyllium Husk Powder, Ground Brown Linseed, Fermented Maize Starch, Salt, Calcium, **Colour: Plain Caramel,** Linseed Fibre, Vitamins (Niacin, Pantothenic Acid, Vitamin B6, Riboflavin, Folic Acid)	Water, Potato Flour, Corn Starch, Tapioca Starch, Sunflower Seeds 4%, Brown Rice Flour, Buckwheat flour, Linseeds 32%, **Thickening Agents (Xanthan Gum, Cellulose,** Agar), Treacle, Millet Seeds 2%, Yeast, Glycerol, Poppy Seeds 1%, Rice Bran, Pea Protein, Rapeseed Oil, Salt, Apple Fibre, Sourdough (Fermented Quinoa, Rice and Maize Flour), Psyllium Husk, Acids (Citric Acid, Malic Acid, Tartaric Acid), **Acidifier (Glucono-Delta-Lactone),** Flour Treatment Agent (Ascorbic Acid)	Water, Tapioca Starch, Potato Starch, Maize Starch, Rapeseed Oil, Yeast, Rice Flour Topping (Water, Rice Flour, Sugar, Potato Starch, Flavouring), Egg White Powder, **Stabiliser: E464,** Vegetable Fibre (Psyllium), Sugar, Fruit Extract (Carob and Apple), Salt, **Humectant: Vegetable Glycerine, Preservatives: Calcium Propionate, Potassium Sorbate,** Rice Flour, Natural Flavouring	Water, Gluten Free Oat Flakes, Sunflower Seeds, Brown Linseeds, Golden Linseeds, Pumpkin Seeds, Millet Seeds, Psyllium Fibre, Milled Brown Linseed, Apple Cider Vinegar, Himalayan Salt
✗	✗	✗	✓

Organic diet

If you suffer from rosacea I believe it is very important for you to choose, whenever possible, organic options. I know there are many sceptical voices when it comes to organic food (I certainly have them in my family), suggesting that these are the same products just labelled as 'organic' (in some countries the term 'organic' is substituted with 'bio' or 'eco') to be more expensive. Well, not quite. Let's first understand what the term 'organic' means in reference to foods.

The 'organic products' indicates the way agricultural products and livestock are grown, raised and processed. Organically produced food is different from mass-farmed food and here is why.

Organic crops have to be grown without any GMOs, pesticides (even small amounts of pesticide residue can be harmful if consumed regularly), synthetic herbicides, or fertilizers which conventional mass farming uses a lot. The substances used for protecting crops and ensuring their potent sizing, attractive colouring etc. penetrate the plants and then we consume those chemicals. In the long term, they affect our gut and liver health and can be responsible for all sorts of modern chronic conditions. In contrast, organic foods aren't contaminated with any dangerous chemical substances that could be harmful to consumers. Organic vegetables and fruit are also fresher than regular, conventional products which are often infused with preservatives to make them last longer. What's more, studies show that organic plant foods have higher value of antioxidants, vitamins and minerals than non-organic options.

Organic livestock means that the livestock raised for meat, eggs, or dairy products has to be raised in conditions compliant with their natural environment, with the ability to graze on pasture. They also need to be fed organic feed and forage, and can't be given any antibiotics or growth hormones. Organic meat and eggs are better because they don't contain harmful substances that potentially mass farming products do but also have a much better nutritional profile- higher Omega3 level, lower Omega6/Omega3 ratio, higher levels of vitamins and minerals and other beneficial substances.

Supporting organic farming is also, I think, the moral thing to do as it promotes animal welfare. It is also better for the environment- uses less energy, pollutes the environment a lot less than conventional farming, increases soil fertility, and reduces soil erosion (in contrast to farming that uses synthetic chemicals).

If you have a garden, I encourage you to plant your favourite vegetables, herbs and fruit trees and create your mini organic heaven. If you have enough space you can even keep chickens for your own organic eggs.

Finding your favourite food substitutions

Eliminating processed foods, sugar, snacks, gluten, etc. from your diet may sound scary to you, especially if you were eating them regularly. And I get it. It wasn't the easiest thing for me either. But changes like that are only distressing at first, and trust me, once we get used to them, they all become our new normal. It is like moving house- at first, you have lots of work to do, then it takes you time to get used to the new layout and where everything lives but eventually, it all becomes normal and familiar to you.

While we transition towards an optimal health diet, we must understand that this process is not only about eliminating unhealthy options like deli meats, alcohol, sweets etc. but about replacing them with healthy and tasty options. It is important we don't feel like we are losing something, so instead we must focus on the variety of options we have. These days, we have access to so many great recipes online and making nutritious meals and snacks that are simple, delicious and healthy, has never been easier. It is important to find an interest (and maybe soon a passion) in healthy meal prep and cooking and use your creativity. You need to feel satisfied with your food to remain on this path, otherwise, you will constantly be tempted to go back to your old eating habits.

Something that I always repeat to my children is that if you don't like some foods, try them in a different configurations. For example, I find boiled or steamed cauliflower dull and I would need to force myself to eat it, but I absolutely love roasted cauliflower seasoned with my favourite spices!

These are examples of my favourite foods substitutions:

- Sweet snacks - fruit like blueberries, black grapes, oranges, wholegrain rice cakes with good-quality nut butter and sliced banana with a pinch of cinnamon, dark chocolate (min 85%).

- Savoury snacks - carrot or celery sticks with hummus, healthy savoury snacks (in the UK we have brands like: Ella's Kitchen, Naked, Ape or Biona, etc. which make healthy but convenient snacks).

- Alcohol- I believe some people drink not for the flavour, but for the relaxing state they can achieve, so why not replace an evening drink with a relaxing bath with Epsom salts, candles and calming music. I personally love this way of 'unwinding';

Dairy- yes or not?

This is a tricky one because the studies are inconclusive about whether dairy is beneficial or not for human health. However, it is confirmed that 65 to 70% of the world's population has some form of lactose (sugar naturally occurring in milk) intolerance. The medical world also noticed a link between dairy consumption and acne, adult acne, eczema and other skin conditions (including rosacea). High dairy consumption is also linked to gut inflammation.

Dr Natasha Campbell-McBride (the GAPs diet founder) believes that the issues people have with commercial dairy come from the fact that all dairy found in the shops is pasteurized. The pasteurisation process deprives milk of the beneficial enzymes that help humans to digest it. She recommends consuming raw milk products instead (often you can buy them directly from your local farmers).

I completely stopped eating dairy in the first 3 months of my rosacea healing diet (when focusing on my gut health) but then gradually started including organic hard cheeses (like cheddar and parmesan) - they are lactose free. I also started consuming raw, unpasteurised butter on a daily basis.

If you don't see any link between dairy consumption and rosacea flare-ups and you decide to continue eating dairy, I recommend choosing organic milk from cows that are free of growth hormones and it contains more Omega-3 fatty acids and conjugated linoleic acid. If you have access to raw organic dairy, that is even better.

Alcohol

Regular alcohol consumption is known to elevate the risk of high blood pressure, cancer, liver disease, stroke and all sorts of gut health issues- including gut dysbiosis and leaky gut. Even a small amount of alcohol is considered as a toxin by our liver and gut. It is also a well-known flare-up trigger for rosacea sufferers. I recommend excluding alcohol completely from your diet and lifestyle while healing from rosacea.

Eating out

A vast amount of the Western society loves eating out and loves food to come all ready to eat. Unfortunately, eating out is problematic, especially in a phase when you are trying to improve your gut and liver health. Why? Because it is important at this stage not to consume any processed food with added synthetic substances and mass farming foods in which many chemicals are used. Most restaurants, pubs and bars (not even mentioning takeaway places) use cheaper, longer-lasting products to ensure cost-effectiveness. Even the most pricey eating places don't guarantee using organic and unprocessed products. When you are eating out you simply don't know what kind of food is being served to you, even if it's cooked to perfection.

When you are coming out of the gut and/or liver healing phase and you moved to a healthy (anti-inflammatory) diet, eating out still shouldn't be something you do often for the same reason.

Although I don't think the occasional (let's say once a week) eating out will do any harm - as long as you're choosing your meals consciously. Do not let the menu (or your companion's food choices) tempt you to go for lots of gluten, starch and sugar. I usually choose something like grilled fish, steak and side vegetables and I avoid any chips, bread, pasta or desserts.

Often people feel that avoiding eating out may affect their social life. If that's the case I highly recommend you start cooking for your friends (or cooking together) and inviting them over for social gatherings with delicious and healthy foods! If you're invited to someone's house, make sure you bring some healthy foods with you (for yourself and others to try). Salads, gluten-free pasta, tacos, soups, stews, curries and nutritious snacks! Party foods can be healthy and the options are limitless... Who knows, maybe you will even inspire others to eat better!

80/20% rule

I am well aware that all my rosacea healing diet suppositions may sound too extreme for you, especially if you are someone who so far has been eating convenience and processed foods regularly. But I would also like to stress that personally, I didn't change my diet overnight. This process happened gradually alongside the growth of my awareness and knowledge. I must say, however, that having rosacea was the best motivation possible for me to improve my diet.

There was a period during my journey (after a couple of months probably) when I became obsessed with eating healthily. I was putting too much pressure and stress upon myself, and that wasn't good for my mental state at all.

Luckily, I learnt about the 80/20% healthy eating rule. It means that as long as we eat a healthy diet 80% of the time, we can afford 20% on 'not great' foods without impacting our health. This rule turned out to be very helpful for me as I stopped feeling guilty about not always eating my ideal diet. That's why I still allow myself homemade pizza (that I love!) once in a while. I will also eat a cake on my kid's birthday (yes- with refined sugar and dairy) and I have ice cream when I'm on holiday and I don't beat myself up for it.

The 80/20 % rule I believe is genius, especially for people who intend to diametrically change their diet. To succeed, we need to feel good about our choices instead of feeling guilty; having a little space for deviation reduces the pressure.

Short-term diets versus long-term habits change

Many people with rosacea have contacted me through my Instagram profile (@alicia.piot), saying that they went on a liver detox program and/or had focused on gut healing and had noticed massive improvements to their skin but then they moved back to their 'normal' eating patterns and rosacea came back. Most people don't understand why and feel very disappointed.

A massive problem with Western society is that many are very short-sighted and always want to take shortcuts.
Quick fixes don't work with rosacea, or any chronic condition really.

Do you think going on liver detox and then returning to all the bad habits, like eating processed foods and takeaways will make your rosacea reverse permanently?

Focusing on gut health, eating lots of gut-healing nutrients, improving your diet for a couple of weeks or even months and as soon as your skin looks better, going back to your previous lifestyle will heal your rosacea?

Sadly, no. If you are to think about quick fixes for rosacea, you will be constantly fluctuating between better skin and flare-ups...

I'm happy to say that today I'm completely rosacea free and I have no doubt that I owe it to a permanent dietary and lifestyle change. I never went back to eating processed foods and takeaways. I never stopped checking the labels and rejecting any foods with synthetic substances. I never stopped eating an organic diet, I never returned to a diet full of gluten and other grains. I simply stuck to an amazing anti-inflammatory diet and choose to look after my gut and liver health on a daily basis. This lifestyle and approach to nutrition are natural and intuitive for me now.

Yes, I know it doesn't help that the modern world promotes fast foods- they are everywhere. The same applies to convenient pre-made and pre-packed options. Gluten is everywhere too- pastries, sandwiches, cakes and pizzas are literally surrounding us... Yet, I want to assure you, once your mindset changes about food and its nutritional value, you will start noticing lots of options for yourself out there. This process of changing your approach to food and not being tempted by foods that are not great for you takes time so be patient. Try to look at things from a long-term perspective, be kind to yourself and remember about the 80%/20% rule ☺

The costs of a healthy diet

Every time I talk to my friends or family about my diet they assume I spend lots of money on food. I am always honest – yes, organic, fresh foods and good ingredients are more expensive and I do spend lots of money on my grocery shopping. But on the other hand, I don't spend any money on alcohol or cigarettes, sweets, cakes, desserts or takeaways and I rarely eat out. I don't over-eat so I don't consume large amounts of food. So overall, do I spend more money eating a healthy, organic and anti-inflammatory diet than when I was eating an ordinary, modern western, convenient and highly processed diet? NO.

My rosacea healing diet steps

Above I tackled the most important dietary topics that relate to rosacea and our optimal health. I hope I managed to increase your awareness when it comes to nutrition and you can now understand how our food choices can affect our health and cause rosacea. In this subchapter, I would like to outline all the steps I did in terms of my diet to reverse my rosacea. This way you can get a sense of how my dietary adjustments looked in practice.

1. In the beginning, I took a gut health test to determine if I had any gut abnormalities, as well as a detailed blood test (I had them both done privately). This was followed by a consultation with a nutritionist and naturopath who advised me on the next steps- the gut healing diet, liver support, supplements and lifestyle.
2. I started a gut-healing diet (this faze lasted about 3 months):
- I avoided high-histamine foods (like chocolate, avocado or tomatoes) and dairy (I have noticed that I am sensitive to high-histamine foods and dairy and experienced rosacea flare-ups after eating them)
- I completely eliminated gluten for 3 months and avoided all the grains (but would occasionally have gluten-free grains like oats, basmati rice or quinoa).
- I avoided other starchy foods (like potatoes).
- I completely eliminated refined sugar, alcohol and any processed foods from my diet.
- I stopped drinking coffee and tea for 3 months and substituted them with herbal teas: mint, nettle, holy basil (Tulsi), turmeric and ginger.

- I was doing intermittent fasting every day.
- I implemented gut-healing foods, such as home-made chicken broth and home-made fermented foods (I took it from the GAPs diet recommendations), which I would eat pretty much every day for 3 months.
- I was taking supplements recommended by my nutritionist (for me they were probiotics matched to my particular gut dysbiosis, fish oil, vitamin D, sodium butyrate, zinc, vitamin B complex, and colostrum); I strongly advise you to test and consult with a health professional first before taking any supplements.
- My liver health tests (included in my blood and urine tests) came back good but I decided to include in my diet liver-supporting foods such as broccoli sprouts, watercress and dark leafy greens, chlorella powder, milk thistle and turmeric (added to my daily smoothie), and dandelion root tea.
- For the first 3 months, my diet mostly consisted of homemade chicken broth, vegetable soups (made with my broth), various organic meat, organic vegetables (mostly cooked), my Rosacea Healing Smoothie (p.77) and herbal teas. Remember every person is different and your gut issues may be different to mine, it may take longer to heal your guts. I believe 3 months is a minimum.

3. After 3 months I started gradually moving to an anti-inflammatory diet (I am still on this diet and planning to continue it forever!)
- Still, there were no heavy processed foods for me (nothing with synthetic substances); yes I always read the labels!
- I continued eating chicken broth at least 3 times a week and regularly consumed fermented foods.

- I started cooking daily, mostly from fresh, basic ingredients; I have learnt to cook easy, simple meals full of nutrients and anti-inflammatory ingredients.
- The base of my diet was vegetables, salads, organic meat, wild fatty sea fish, lots of dark green leaves, berries, seeds and nuts.
- I still avoided gluten (but I would have it occasionally).
- I went back to eating grains (only in moderation though) but I switched to gluten-free options of bread, flour and pasta- only with good natural ingredients and without synthetic additives in the composition.
- I ate starchy foods only in moderation (rice, gluten-free pasta, oats, quinoa, buckwheat and potatoes).

My new diet (anti-inflammatory diet) proportions for healing rosacea:

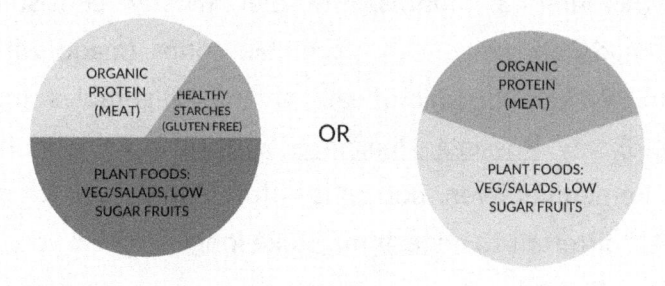

ORGANIC PROTEIN (MEAT) | HEALTHY STARCHES (GLUTEN FREE) | PLANT FOODS: VEG/SALADS, LOW SUGAR FRUITS

OR

ORGANIC PROTEIN (MEAT) | PLANT FOODS: VEG/SALADS, LOW SUGAR FRUITS

My old diet (modern diet) proportions:

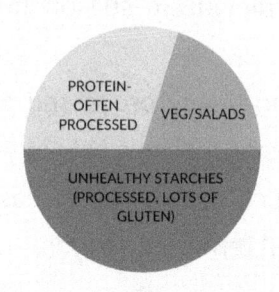

PROTEIN- OFTEN PROCESSED | VEG/SALADS | UNHEALTHY STARCHES (PROCESSED, LOTS OF GLUTEN)

- Every day, I used plenty of healthy anti-inflammatory spices and herbs like turmeric, ginger, garlic, oregano, basil, parsley, chives, mint, nigella seeds etc.
- I started eating a good amount of healthy Omega3 fats. Around four times a week, I would eat fatty sea fish: wild salmon, cod, sardines, herrings or mackerel. Every day, I used cold-pressed flaxseed and olive oil to increase my healthy oils intake, and occasionally I also used coconut and avocado oil.
- I was still avoiding refined sugars (I would only have it occasionally, but never as processed food; for example, I would eat a small piece of homemade cake when I was visiting family or a friend).
- I still didn't eat dairy other than hard cheeses like cheddar and parmesan (they are lactose-free) and raw butter.
- I returned to drinking green tea and good-quality caffeine-free organic coffee (as I don't feel great after consuming caffeine) once my face was rosacea-free. Coffee and green tea are very high in many amazing compounds that contribute to our health, and they actually fight inflammation.
- Whenever possible I always buy organic food.
- I continued with intermittent fasting on most days.
- I didn't drink any alcohol for another 3 months and after that time I would occasionally have a glass of red wine (no more than once a week); small amounts of red wine has anti-inflammatory properties due to its high levels of plant nutrients called polyphenols.

Following the above protocol, my skin started to improve after just several weeks (on a gut and liver-healing diet). Five to six months later (eating an anti-inflammatory diet) my face was completely rosacea free.

All this time I was also learning a lot about nutrition. I wanted to know and understand it all myself. I kept reading books and listening to podcasts. I was discovering an unlimited number of anti-inflammatory recipes for daily meals, snacks, party foods, etc. I spent time figuring out how to cook simple, wholesome, delicious meals, that made me feel satisfied so I no longer crave rubbish foods any more. I also learnt how not to become obsessed with healthy eating but made it an instinctive choice. I learnt how to balance my new diet with my family's preferences, and how not to feel like a victim of any 'healthy' regime.

Of course, this is all a topic for another book, but I just want to let you know that eating a healthy diet gets easier and more intuitive with time, and please don't ever beat yourself up for finding it difficult at the beginning of the transition.

I believe the journey to healing rosacea is more about learning about nutrition and a healthy lifestyle and re-evaluating our habits rather than forcing ourselves to live the ways we don't like. Today I have no doubt this was the key to my success story – I didn't only make a short-term change to beat the inflammation in my skin, I made the permanent shifts in my diet, my lifestyle and really, my whole outlook on wellbeing.

My favourite anti-inflammatory foods which I include in my meals:

PROTEINS	- Organic meat - Fatty fish: wild salmon, mackerel, herring, sardines, seafood - Eggs - Dried green lentils (soaked and then cooked)
FATS	- Olive oil - Flaxseed oil - Avocado oil - Chia seeds - Flaxseeds - Walnuts - Almonds - Sunflower seeds - Sesame seeds - Pumpkin seeds
FRUITS	- All berries especially blueberries - Pomegranate - Red grapes - Oranges - Coconut
VEGETABLES	- Broccoli - Cabbage - Cauliflower - Pak choi - Tomatoes - Carrot - Cucumber - Leek - Courgette - Beetroot
HERBS, SPICES, GREEN LEAVES	- Spices: ginger, garlic, onion, turmeric, thyme, black cumin - Herbs: oregano, parsley, nettle, rosemary, basil, peppermint, thyme, sage, chives, green onions, dill - Green leaves: watercress, rocket (arugula), pea shoots, spinach, all lettuces with dark leaves, broccoli sprouts
STARCHY FOODS (small amounts)	- Quinoa - Millet - Brown and wild rice - Buckwheat - Wholegrain oats (gluten free) - Sweet potatoes - Potatoes
BEVERAGES	- Water - Herbal teas: mint, holly, basil, nettle, ginger and turmeric
SWEETNERS (minimal amounts)	- Raw Honey - Maple Syrup - Date syrup - Dates

Anti-inflammatory herbs and spices that help to heal rosacea:

Include them in your everyday diet to heal Rosacea
(fresh or dried)

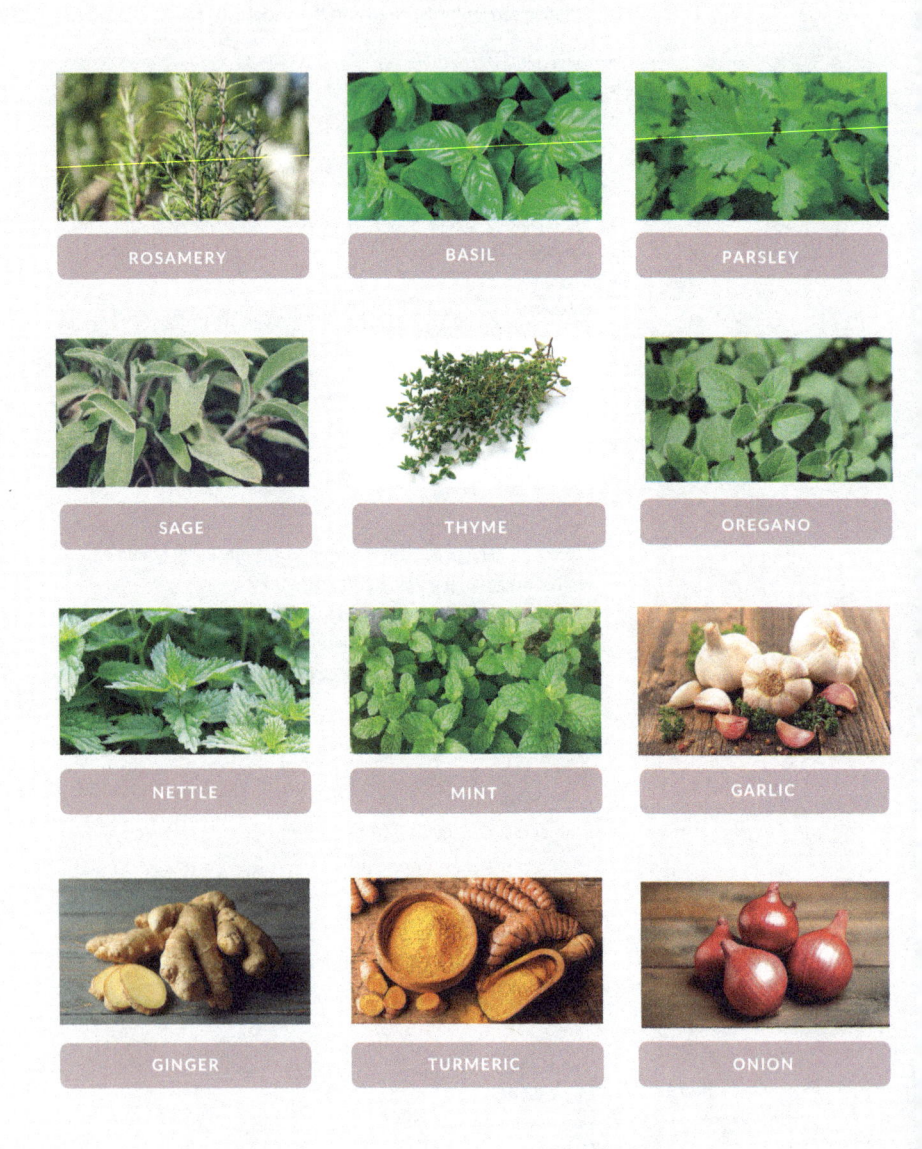

ROSAMERY	BASIL	PARSLEY
SAGE	THYME	OREGANO
NETTLE	MINT	GARLIC
GINGER	TURMERIC	ONION

Frozen Blueberry Rosacea Healing Smoothie

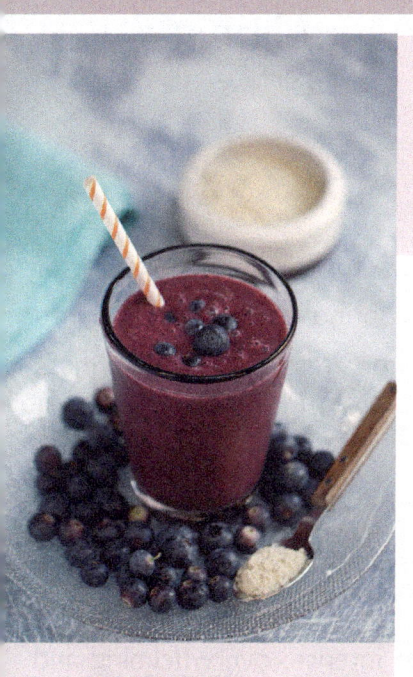

PREP TIME: LESS THAN 10 MIN

SERVES 2 BIG GLASSES

INGREDIENTS

1 unripe banana (yellow with a bit of green)
3/4 cups of frozen blueberries
1-2 cups of water (depending on the consistency you like)
2 tablespoons of flaxseeds
1 tablespoon of chlorella powder
1 teaspoon of milk thistle
1 tablespoon of raw honey (optional)
1 tablespoon of psyllium husk (a great source of fibre)
1 tablespoon of dried turmeric + pinch of black pepper

DIRECTION

Pop it all into your high-speed blender and enjoy as a very healthy drink or plate it up as a smoothie bowl. For this option simply decorate with other fruits, nuts, chia seeds and/or sugar-free, gluten-free granola!

NOTES

Unripe bananas are a great source of resistant starch which feeds our good gut bacteria.

Freezing blueberries increases the concertation of anthocyanins, which are natural anti-inflammatory agents.

Raw honey (not pasteurised) is full of inflammation-fighting antioxidants and has anti-bacterial properties.

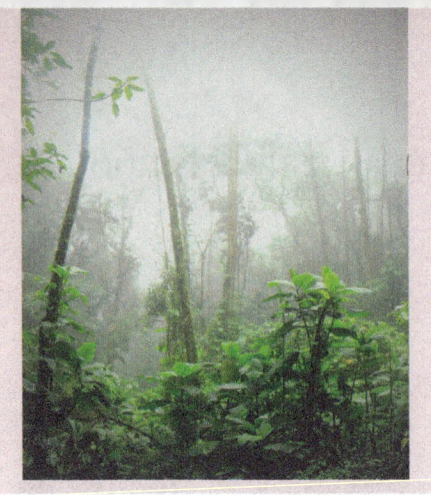

09

Stress management and emotional wellbeing

Chronic stress is another indicated factor for the occurrence of chronic inflammation. When stress hormones are released into our bodies, they provoke inflammatory responses in our mass cells. If we feel tense all the time those hormones constantly circulate in our systems.

Even though living conditions, abundance and world safety are better than they have ever been before, humanity's stress levels are at a peak. Life these days is so intense, overwhelming and pressurising on every level. We've reached a point where the number of stimulants (technology, media, social media, accessible excitements), social and economic pressures, things we must achieve, solve, deal with – all of it is just too much for our nervous systems. Panic attacks, anxiety, nervous breakdowns, addictions, depression, and chronic inflammatory conditions are more common now than ever before. We simply cannot stop stressing and worrying.

Obviously, I always knew stress wasn't good for me and I was aware I was stressing and worrying too much. I would always imagine all possible future problems and used to overthink the negative events from the past. I would always focus my attention on the dark side of reality, things that I am lacking, adversities and negativity. As you can imagine that was making me unhappy and overwhelmed. I can't explain why, but I always believed I didn't have another choice and that my stress was a natural and normal response to everything that was happening around me. It was not until I realised that stress affects me much more than just mentally and emotionally. It affects my physical health, trashes my gut microbes and causes inflammation in my body. Only when I learnt that rosacea may be an effect of my chronic stress, I felt motivated to do something about it.

I decided to begin a personal growth journey. The main purpose was to be able to manage my stress and anxiety and try to be more joyful and positive. Of course, I knew that stress is an inseparable part of life, and we can't always avoid it. But what I have discovered during my journey is that if we make an effort, we can actually find peace inside us, we can learn to trust the universe and we can go through life more smoothly. I discovered that we have a choice, and we can intentionally choose a calmer life.

As it turned out, I actually had a habit of cultivating stress and negative emotions and I used to overthink stuff that I had no influence over. On top of that, I was never giving myself time to unwind; I didn't appreciate time for myself. Back in the day, I rarely allowed myself time to take breaks from hectic family life. I didn't appreciate the importance of being just with myself. I used to always put my own needs last behind my family's (but at the same time, I would consider myself a victim of this). Occasionally, whenever I had some free time, I would choose socialising, going out for a drink with a friend, watching a Netflix series or would scroll through social media. My breaks were never restorative and calming for me; rather they stimulated and distracted me more. Even when I felt overwhelmed, I would never consider going for a walk on my own or taking myself for a weekend away. That would be something beyond my consideration.

Thanks to rosacea, I realised how important it is to tackle my stress, daily pressures and anxieties. Soon I also understood that it is not a change that can be made in one day. Having the right intention is the first step, but learning to manage the stress takes time. It is a pretty long process of working regularly with various relaxation techniques. To be effective, the process requires consistency and your full commitment.

Therefore, I decided to try something new. I started having 'me time' – quality time in which I would be on my own, free from any pressures or daily chores. Every day I would log off social media and any other stimulants to indulge myself in various relaxing techniques.

There are many ways you can intentionally find and organise quality 'me time'. My favourites are during the early mornings, before the rest of my family wakes up, between 5 and 7am. But the evenings can also bring a perfect quiet and relaxing space for healing practices like meditation, affirmations, gratitude and visualisations.

My favourite practices that help me to lower my stress level, relax and unwind daily:

01 GUIDED MEDITATIONS

I absolutely love these meditations which are led by a narrator who guides you through. You will be instructed on your posture, breathing, visualisations and mental images. Guided meditations usually concentrate on particular topics like stress, anxiety, forgiveness, body healing etc. Whatever problem you want to work on, you will find suitable audio-guided meditations for it. You can find them on streaming platforms like YouTube, iTunes or Spotify. I encourage you to be intuitive when choosing your guided mediation, you know best what you need at the moment and what would serve you the most.

Remember that it is also important to find the right narrator for you (for example, I only like meditations guided by female voices). I usually practice 10 to 15 minutes of meditation a day during 'me time'.

02 GRATITUDE PRACTICE

It is simply listing the aspects or things in your life for which you feel thankful. When I first came across the idea of daily gratitude, it sounded very naive to me. But soon I learnt that science, psychology, and neurology all confirm that regular gratitude practice significantly increases the level of "happy hormones" in our systems and makes us feel more fulfilled and content with our lives.

Psychology indicates that directing your attention on the good aspects, things and people in your life, can give us sense of abundance and satisfaction.

To practice gratitude, all you need is a peaceful couple minutes a day, ideally some paper and a pen. You can do it at any convenient time. In the morning, before bed, during your lunch break – anytime is good to express appreciation. Personally, I like practicing gratitude first thing in the morning, right before my morning meditation, as it always sets a positive and uplifting tone for my whole day.

Every day, I write down five things for which I am thankful. Sometimes they are little things, like a refreshing shower, or they are significant, like healthy children. Whenever something I am grateful for comes to my mind, I write it down. Thanks to this simple technique I have realised how many blessings I have in my life that I wasn't noticing before; I used to take them for granted. Gratitude practice helped me to overcome negativity and a complaining attitude, and it simply made me more satisfied about my life.

03 POSITIVE AFFIRMATIONS

I cannot recommend them enough. Affirmations are positive statements that are supposed to be repeated every day in order to replace any negative thoughts and beliefs. Our brains and nervous systems are fascinating mechanisms and it turns out that what we continuously hear or experience we believe to be true.

Our childhoods have the biggest impact on our perspectives of reality because we absorb most opinions and attitudes subconsciously.

But luckily, **affirmations have the power to change our negative patterns and massively improve our quality of life.** Thanks to affirmations I managed to work through so many issues of mine. Stress, negativity, low self-esteem, anxiety, loneliness and even things like being disorganised and always late. Affirmations have transformed me into a much more relaxed, trusting, and happier person. I believe affirmations are something everyone should practice for their own benefit. Personally, I am a big fan of Louise Hay's audio affirmations (you can find them on YouTube) and her affirmation cards. But I also listen to various audio affirmations and repeat them after the narrator. There are lots of audio affirmations to find on YouTube and Spotify. You can also note your favourite affirmations down and read them out loud every day. Some people like repeating their affirmations in front of the mirror. For the best results it is important to stick to the ones that resonate with us the most and work with them consistently and regularly.

My favourite affirmations:

Everything is ok in my world.
I am safe, calm and at peace.
I am enough.
I love myself and my life.
I already have everything I need to be happy.
I have a beautiful life.
I can solve any problem.
I have inner calm and I can turn towards it every time I'm in need.
I have loving and respectful relationships with others.
I am doing the best I can, and it is always enough.
I am on the right path.
I am healing.

04 MINDFULNESS

Simply speaking, mindfulness means being present in the moment and concentrating only on the 'here' and 'now'. I think 'mindfulness' is just a big word for going back to the simplicity of living. Simplicity, that soothes our nerves and brings clarity and joy. When we are mindful, we don't think about the past, we don't analyse events, we don't spend time judging others and we don't multitask. We are taking the 'here' and 'now' slowly, with appreciation, full attention, and we are experiencing it with all our senses.

Therefore, mindfulness is a highly effective tool to bring peace and balance to our minds. These days, all the wellbeing professionals, therapists and life-coaches recognise the massive benefits from practicing mindfulness. I see a significant difference in myself since I've worked on being more mindful in everyday life. Thanks to this, I understand that I don't need to multitask, rush, be connected to all the possible sources or devices, and I can just enjoy my here and now; this approach is actually very beneficial for my mental health.

How do I practice mindfulness?
- I disconnect from social media on the weekends, and switch off the internet on my phone after 8pm until 9 the next morning.
- Every day I go for a walk in nature without looking at my phone; I try not to think about anything, I just indulge myself in observing the sky, listening to the birds, touching

the leaves, or sometimes I even walk bare foot on the grass. I immerse myself in the moment.
- I remind myself regularly of my intention to stop ruminating over past events, thinking and overthinking things that have gone wrong, or people who hurt me in the past. I know it won't make any difference anymore, and that I am taking a joy away from myself of being in the present moment.
- I cultivate doing one task at a time, even the simplest things like eating, cleaning the house or playing with the children. I know we all feel pressure to multitask and be extra productive, but you know what, I'd rather be happy, healthy and at peace than extra-productive.

On top of all the above daily calming practices, I also regularly:

- Practice yoga (I attend yoga classes two times per week and practice twice on my own at home).
- Spend as much time outdoors as I can. During the weekends and holidays, I choose to spend time in nature rather than busy shopping malls or going away for city breaks. Being surrounded by nature soothes my nerves like nothing else.
- Practice relaxing breathing techniques when I feel overwhelmed. There are many types, you can find instructions online but the simplest one is to take a deep full inhale for four seconds and give a voiced exhale for eight seconds. I repeat this at least four times.
- Journal- whenever I feel overwhelmed with life, and I need to take the burden off.

I have also started paying attention to what kind of content I am watching and reading and the people with whom I surround myself. I have noticed that I always absorb the energy that is around me and if it's negative, I soon begin to feel upset, agitated and overwhelmed. Therefore, I stopped watching daily news (which in the past, made me believe that we live in a bad and scary world), brutal or very upsetting movies and TV shows with lots of negative energy. I also stopped reading crime books. Finally, I avoid meeting up with people who always complain, gossip, judge others, who swear a lot or who are always grumpy and unhappy. I simply began to make conscious choices about the energy I am inviting in to my life, and I must say that this approach really contributes to my emotional stability.

Options for daily relaxation and emotional healing:

MEDITATION

JOURNALING

GENTLE YOGA PRACTICE

WALKING IN NATURE

GARDENING

PAPER-PRINT BOOK READING

DANCING WHEN NO ONE WATCHES

CALM BATH SOAK

QUIET CREATIVE TIME: PAINTING, COLOURING, KNITTING ETC.

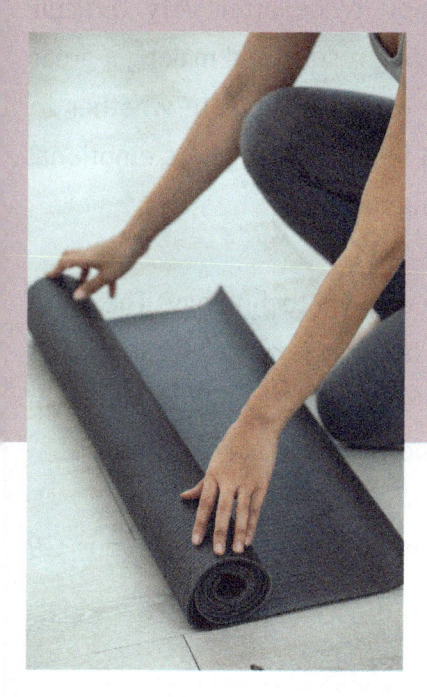

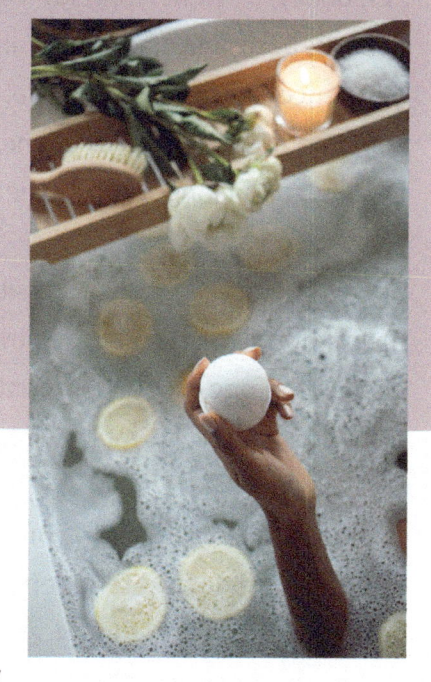

Therapy

Mental health and emotional wellbeing should always be our priority regardless of our skin condition. But it is also worth realising that depression, chronic stress and anxieties not only affect how we feel emotionally but can also cause gut health issues (like gut dysbiosis) and start inflammation within our bodies.

Sometimes the relaxing and self-healing practices I mentioned above are not enough and despite our efforts, we can not find emotional peace and stress/anxiety relief. This especially applies to people who carry a lot of burdens and past traumas can still affect their mental wellbeing. In these cases, I am a big advocate for reaching for professional help and going to therapy.

Personally, I went through therapy twice after very difficult periods, both times achieving amazing results and making a great difference in my everyday life. If you ever hesitate whether to start therapy, I highly recommend you give it a go, as emotional healing goes a long way with healing rosacea.

Today, therapy is easily accessible also via technology. There are many portals that you review hundreds of counsellors and choose the one most appropriate for you. You can also see them from the comfort of your own home via Zoom or Facetime.

If money is an issue for you, remember you can ask your GP (primary care doctor) for a referral.

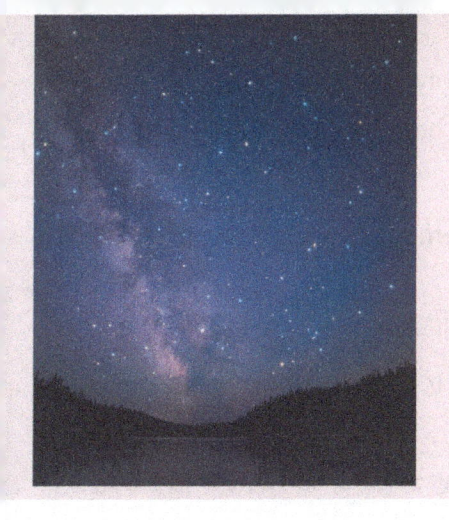

10
Healthy sleep pattern

I was always aware that healthy sleep is important, but I hadn't realised that regular sleep loss can actually activate inflammation markers in our systems and cause cell damage. Poor sleep turns out to have a major effect on inflammation in our bodies and is linked to all sorts of inflammatory conditions. It affects our central nervous system, particularly the stress response system, which helps us to regulate our stress levels. Not enough sleep or sleep that is too disturbed can increase our stress levels and make us more vulnerable when dealing with life. As we already know, stress hormones trigger inflammatory mediators in our bodies. If you want to reverse your rosacea, looking after your sleep hygiene is crucial.

Rosacea first appeared on my face when my little boy was around ten months old. I hadn't really slept properly ever since he was born. When I realised the importance of my sleep, I decided to make some changes. I had a fantastic consultation with a naturopath who gave me lots of valuable advice on how to improve my sleep pattern. Based on her advice and my own research, I implemented new bedtime rules that helped me to sleep much better. This not only contributed to my rosacea healing, but I simply felt so much healthier and more energised.

My sleep improvement steps included:

- Practicing daily relaxations like meditation, mindfulness and walks in nature to help me to de-stress and calm my busy mind.
- Improving my diet by avoiding sugars, caffeine and alcohol as well as processed foods
- Supplementing magnesium (I take it in the evening).
- Going to bed early (before 10pm) and getting up before 6am. I am very consistent with my night-time routine and I continue to do the same during the holidays and weekends.
- No blue light devices (phones, iPads) for at least an hour before bedtime.
- A quiet time before bedtime (relaxing bath, meditation, time for prayer- any calming techniques are very helpful here).
- A completely dark space at night or a red/orange/yellow night light.

I believe that it is so important for any rosacea sufferer (or anyone with other inflammatory conditions) to start appreciating the quality of their sleep.

Every morning we should feel well rested and energised and if we don't, we should start looking at ways to improve our sleep.

I have also noticed that **good sleep plays a massive role in maintaining a healthy diet and lifestyle.** When we are overtired, we tend to reach for easy and convenient food and we lack motivation for physical activity or even relaxing practices.

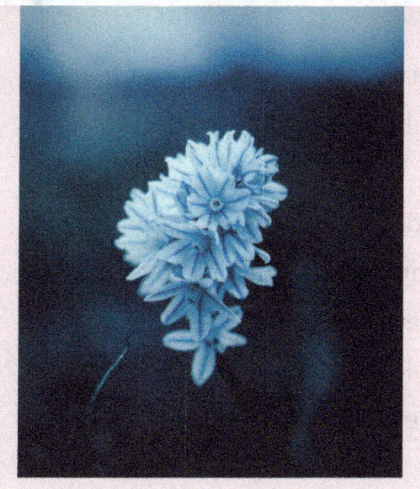

11

Sensible approach to over-the-counter medications and antibiotics

We already know that taking antibiotics not only kills the bad bacteria we may have, but they also trash the friendly and beneficial microbes that our bodies need to work properly. Since learning about gut dysbiosis and its big impact on all sorts of chronic inflammation occurring in the body, I started being much more cautious when it comes to antibiotic therapy. I have already mentioned that my rosacea appeared after one year of taking antibiotics frequently for my ear infections and then mastitis (breast gland infection, when I was breastfeeding). I knew that wasn't the only reason, but I am now convinced it had a big impact on the imbalance that occurred in my system.

Of course, sometimes there are some obvious bacterial conditions in which taking antibiotics is necessary. However, now I understand that we should take good-quality probiotics for at least three months after we complete the prescribed course of antibiotics in order to rebuild the healthy microbes in our digestive systems. It is inexplicable for me that conventional-medicine doctors never advised me to supplement with probiotics after completing a course of antibiotics.

Something that I have also learnt was that not only antibiotics cause a change in our microbiome but so do other medications.

Not all meds have yet been studied from this perspective but there is increasing evidence showing that all meds affect our gut and tax our liver- this includes over-the-counter medications like painkillers, sore throat pastilles, cold and flu meds, etc. Therefore, it is important to stay cautious when it comes to taking any meds.

I have happily noticed that ever since my rosacea disappeared as a result of a good diet, healthy lifestyle and my improved general health, I hardly ever get sick. I don't get headaches anymore and I don't have period pains that previously used to bother me greatly. Simply speaking, I don't need those over-the-counter medications on which I used to rely. There are many natural alternatives, for example, for colds I use ginger, turmeric and propolis in my hot drink or in my meals and I find them highly effective. It is worth remembering that all over-the-counter meds may help to relieve our symptoms (as opposed to the cause) in the short-term, but a regular intake has potentially harmful long-term effects. My rosacea journey has taught me to think about my health in the long-term and to make conscious choices on every occasion.

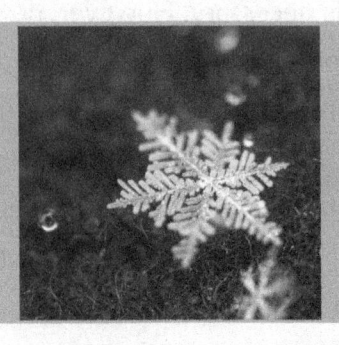

"Taking antibiotics not only kills the bad bacteria we may have, but they also trash the friendly and beneficial microbes that our bodies need to work properly."

ALICIA PIOT

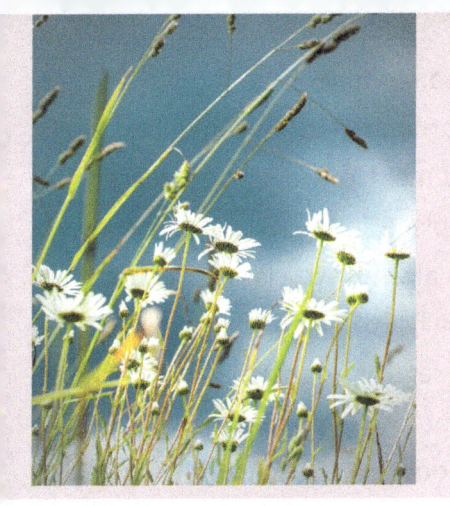

12

Physical activity and rosacea

I was never too interested in sport or exercise. I always had to force myself to work out and it was easy for me to find an excuse not to do it especially since becoming a mother. I must admit, I had abandoned physical exercise for a long time. But then rosacea came into my life and as I explored the topic of body inflammation, I came across many studies indicating that the **lack of or too little physical activity contributes to systemic inflammations, whereas regular exercise helps to keep inflammation in check**. When our muscles work, anti-inflammatory molecules are released into our systems. Only 20 to 30 minutes of physical activity a day starts this positive process in our bodies.

Well, I thought to myself, finally I have the right motivation to start working out. I just had to find the type of workout that I would enjoy. Something that I had tried before and liked was yoga, so I decided to give it a go again. I turned on a 30-minute yoga flow video on YouTube and for the first time ever, I did the complete yoga practice. I felt amazing afterwards – relaxed and settled but energised at the same time. The boost of high vibrational waves that came through not only my body, but through me as a whole surprised me. Now, over two years later, yoga has found its permanent place in my life. I practice it a minimum of four times a week, I attend two classes and practice it at home as well (which are usually 20-minute practices). Today, with no hesitation, I can tell that regular yoga practice has played a massive part in the process of not only my rosacea healing, but in my general fitness and body strengthening. Yoga also contributes to improvement of my mental health and helps me to manage daily stress. Thanks to yoga, I began to feel stronger in every aspect of myself.

There's a wide variety of yoga styles to choose from such as ashtanga, hatha, kundalini, vinyasa, restorative yoga and many more. They are all based on the same foundations but have different dynamics. I encourage you to explore the options to see which one will suit you the most. The two styles I love are vinyasa flow and hatha yoga. Be aware that not every teacher will be suitable for you, just listen to your gut instinct in what works the best for you.

Regular yoga practice increases stamina and strengthens our muscles, joints and ligaments. It helps to detoxify our bodies from toxins, and regulates our glands and hormones.
Practising yoga also supports our nervous systems, improves our immunity, and even slows down the ageing process.

Yoga also helps to relieve tension and reduce everyday stress levels. It is just the perfect exercise for any inflammatory condition sufferer.

On top of yoga, my naturopath advised me to take daily fast walks (a little bit like if you are in a rush). "A fast walk is effective physical exercise as well," she said. I hadn't known that, and realised it was a great way to exercise especially while walking the dog. My husband and I used to always argue about who would take the dog for a walk and now I do it with pleasure as a part of keeping fit. I take my dog to the local parks and woods which is also a bonus as I get to spend time in nature.

Of course, there are so many different sports you can choose from: swimming, running, gym, boxing, cycling, home workout, etc which can get you moving. You don't need to stick to a particular exercise, it is actually good to mix them up. But if you're not a big fan of working out, it may take time to incorporate regular physical activity into your life. Taking small steps but being consistent is always the best way to go. You can start with only 20mins of exercises a day and then gradually increase it (or not). Trust me, it is not that hard- you don't need to run marathons to implement the regular activity in your lifestyle. As I said before, even fast walking counts!

You've probably heard the recommendation to avoid physical activity as getting hot can cause your rosacea to flare. If you think short-term, yes exercising may make your face redder but thinking long-term, it is a crucial element in reversing rosacea. Daily physical activity has countless health benefits but what interests us the most, is that it reduces body inflammations, regulates the digestive system and supports your gut health. Sweating also helps your liver to detoxify. On top of that, regular exercise can help you to sleep better and lower your stress level.

13

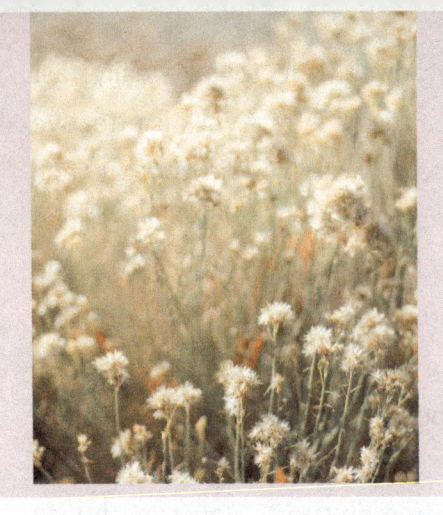

Rosacea skincare

I am honestly convinced that the most amazing (or the most expensive) skincare can not heal rosacea itself, because it isn't a skin condition - it only shows through the skin. Rosacea is connected to the systemic imbalance and that's what we should focus on if we want to heal our skin.

But to say that I also want to stress that the right skincare and conscious approach to choosing all your cosmetics can definitely help your skin (and your body) to heal.

Throughout my rosacea healing journey, I have learnt that the most gentle products are the best options for inflamed skin. In the beginning, I used way too many cosmetics (ones that targeted rosacea) and they only aggravated my skin. Once I started learning about inflammation, I realised that all those products contain lots of chemicals, preservatives and other harsh ingredients that absorb into the skin and through it to our systems, potentially congesting our liver and increasing inflammation.

Since I came to understand chronic inflammatory conditions, my approach towards my wellbeing changed. In line with my dietary and lifestyle modifications, my new skincare routine transformed into being very gentle, natural and minimalistic.

The steps I implemented into my rosacea-curing skincare:

- I stopped using and trying numerous products. I realised I was overwhelming my skin with too many cosmetics. I stopped using exfoliators, facemasks, toners, day-and-night creams and serums.

- I bought one gentle facewash and a skin barrier repair moisturiser, both dedicated to very sensitive and damaged skin. On top of that, I purchased organic 100% rose water, powdered pure hyaluronic acid and pure Vitamin C powder. They all work to soothe sore skin, prone to redness.

- I washed my face with facewash before going to bed, then sprayed it with rosewater and patted it dry with a cotton pad. Then I applied a thin layer of barrier repair moisturiser.

- In the morning, I only washed my face with water, dried it with a clean towel and applied rosewater mixed with hyaluronic acid – sometimes I added a little bit of Vitamin C powder. I mixed it in the palm of my washed hand each time and then applied it on my skin.

- I started avoiding any sort of liquid foundations as they are usually full of awful ingredients. I substituted them with 100% natural mineral powder foundations (made of only natural compositions) and mineral concealer for redness and blemishes. I would occasionally use mineral bronzer and mascara as well. As my skin improved massively, I was confident to not wear make-up every day.

- I stopped using any chemical sun creams as again- they contain many hash ingredients; instead, I started using mineral sun cream with a good natural composition but only when the sun was strong and I was staying outdoors for a long time. Most of the time, when my skin was inflamed I was choosing to shade my face with a sunhat as I noticed my skin doesn't tolerate sun creams very well.

- I was having regular baths with Dead Sea or Epsom salts which are rich in minerals and have antiseptic and detoxing properties. I would happily dip or wash my face in the bath water each time I had my bath; for the extra detoxing effect it is advised to add a couple of spoonfuls of baking powder into the water and/or apple cider vinegar.

- As well as my skincare, I started to pay attention to the composition of all my hygiene products like deodorants (avoiding any containing aluminium), shampoos and body washes. There are many great, natural options to choose from, made without any harsh or harmful ingredients. I stopped using any body lotions and substituted them with coconut oil.

- I also started paying attention to all my home cleaning products and would buy the eco-friendly ones with the most natural compositions. I stopped using perfumes, scented candles and air fresheners, as they release toxins into the air which we then breathe in.

As you can see, my skincare has transformed to become very minimalist, and I believe this is the best way to go with not only rosacea but any kind of inflammatory condition.

If you believe my attitude is too extreme, and you love testing new cosmetics think again about your liver (and whole body health really) and your daily exposure to colorants, artificial additives (like preservatives), perfumes, mercury, dioxins, and other harmful ingredients in our food, care and household products, not even mentioning air pollution. Having to deal with rosacea may be the best motivation for you to start making conscious choices also when it comes to your skincare.

Laser treatment for rosacea

I had never tried any laser treatments for rosacea as I heard numerous stories about how it worsened rosacea symptoms for many people, not even to mention the pain and stress that came with it.

When I think about laser treatments in regards to rosacea I can't even understand how they could possibly help, since rosacea is not a skin condition. I imagine the only situation they can show a positive effect, is when the cause for your skin condition is an overgrown population of Demodex mites, but then Soolanra cream should be at least as effective!

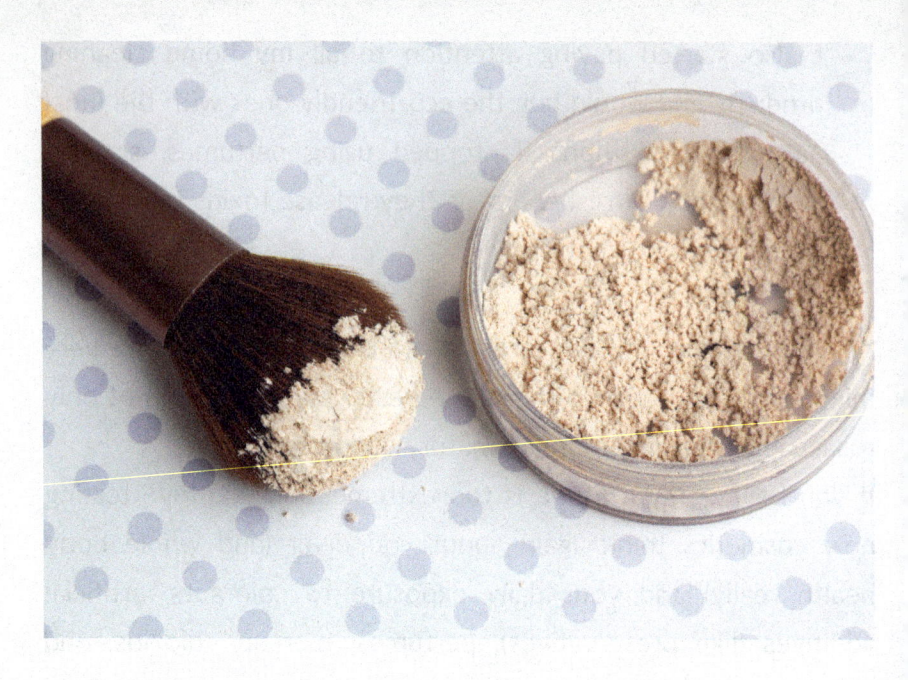

Mineral makeup for covering rosacea

Mineral makeup is a great option for covering acne, rosacea, psoriasis and all sorts of redness. It has great coverage and if applied right- is completely invisible (that's why mineral makeup is a great option for men too).

Mineral powder foundations and concealers are made without parabens, binders, fillers, talc, mineral oil, alcohol, preservatives, and fragrances - all the nasty stuff that actually can increase inflammation in the skin; instead, they contain minerals that are actually beneficial and soothing for the skin.

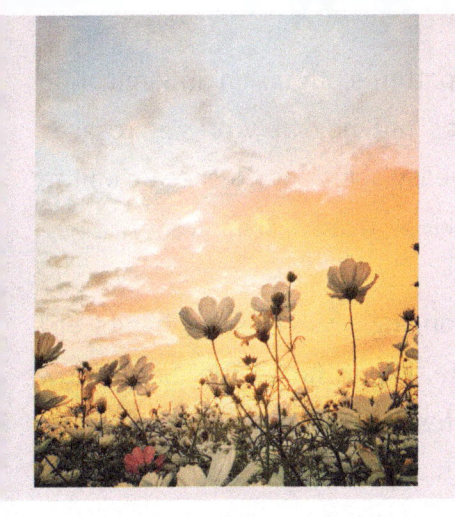

14

The summary of my rosacea healing journey

I have pretty much turned my life around to clear rosacea but I have no regrets. I changed my diet, improved my sleeping patterns, started working out regularly and continuously worked upon reducing my stress levels. I won't lie – it wasn't always easy to change old habits and beliefs for new healthier ones. But my determination and hard work have paid off. Day after day my skin became increasingly clearer and five to six months later, I noticed I had rosacea-free skin.

You know how conventional medicine doctors say you cannot ever reverse rosacea; you can only go into remission and have better or worse moments? I disagree with this. I believe that making permanent diet and lifestyle improvements is the key to saying "goodbye" to rosacea forever. By using word 'permanent' I mean that it can only be a mindset change that will allow you to fully heal rosacea. If I only changed my diet for 3 months and then went back to old eating habits, I'm convinced that my skin would worsen again. I know so many people who went on restrictive diet programs for 3 months to heal their rosacea and their symptoms improved massively; but soon after they went back to their previous eating patterns, the skin inflammation started coming back. Well, that's not how it works – rosacea doesn't like short-term, quick or easy solutions. Rosacea came to your life to encourage you to make permanent changes.

But please, don't think that changing your existing habits will remove enjoyment from your life. No, in fact, I feel better now than ever since I improved my lifestyle. These changes I made in order to beat rosacea – a better diet, regular physical activity and daily stress management – have become a new normal for me and they all make me feel great. I consider this as my big personal success. I have never looked back at my old lifestyle, and I truly believe that's why rosacea hasn't come back.

Now, I look at my experience with rosacea to be my blessing. My face had to become red and inflamed for me to start nurturing my health. Without it, I know I wouldn't have found any motivation to make such radical changes in my eating and living habits. I learnt about chronic inflammation, gut and liver health, and this knowledge seems to be making a huge difference in my own and my family's wellbeing. Thanks to rosacea, I am cultivating this new lifestyle that not only makes me feel healthy and physically stronger but also has massively improved my mental health.

I hope this book has inspired you to reflect on what your skin is trying to communicate to you. You need to think about and nurture your body. Human bodies are amazing holistic creations where all the elements work in very sophisticated and connected ways. Once you realise that, you have a big chance to get to grips with your chronic skin condition.

There's no quick fix to rosacea, there's no effective medication or treatment. But my example shows that there is a long-term solution which we can achieve with permanent diet and lifestyle improvements. I do not doubt that you can overcome your rosacea too by addressing your own systemic imbalances, gut abnormalities and/or liver congestion, stress and other potential factors.

My Rosacea Healing Steps:

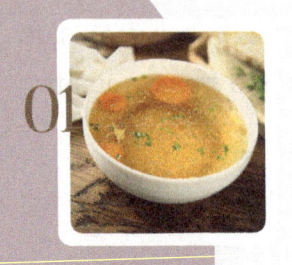

01 Following a gut-healing and liver-supporting diet strictly for 3 months

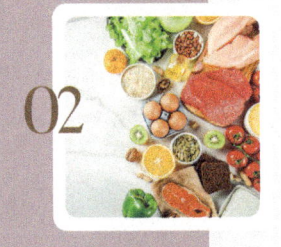

02 After 3 months: gradual transition to an anti-inflammatory diet

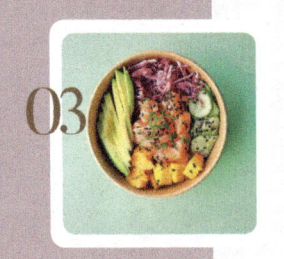

03 Eating an anti-inflammatory diet from now on

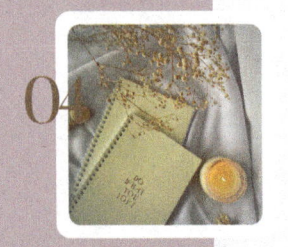

04 Introducing relaxation techniques to my daily routine

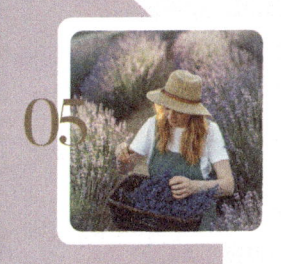

05 Avoiding negativity in my life and concentrating on the positives

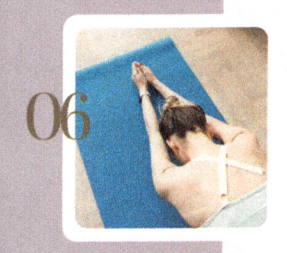

06 Daily physical activity

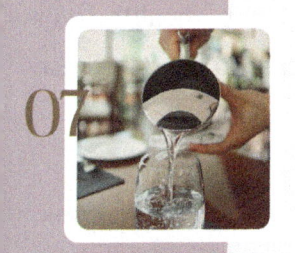

07 Making conscious choices regarding my cosmetics, food and the environment I am living in

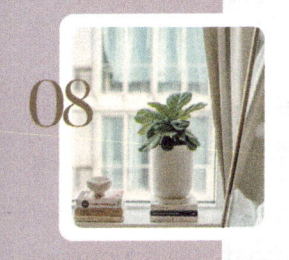

08 Prioritising my sleep

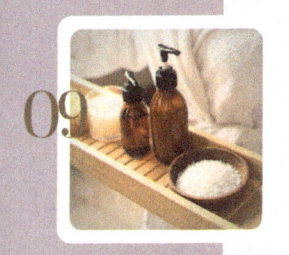

09 Reducing my skincare to the bare minimum and selecting cosmetics with natural composition

To end this book, I would like to give you, my reader and fellow rosacea sufferer, a few hints regarding your own battle with this inflammatory skin condition:

- Think about your rosacea as a manifestation of your inner body imbalance. There is a lot of sense behind rosacea. I encourage you to start learning about and nurturing your own health.

- Think about systemic inflammation, gut health (gut microbiome, leaky gut, SIBO) and liver health. All these turned out to be an answer to my rosacea.

- Reflect on your diet and lifestyle after reading this book. What are you doing right already and what could you do better?

- Remember that changing old eating and living habits requires time, adjustment and learning new ways. Don't beat yourself up that you are unable to go fully gluten-free within one day if previously your diet was based on wheat. Give yourself time, love and compassion.

- If medical doctors are unable to help you with rosacea, this doesn't mean there is nobody to support you in this journey and that there is nothing you can do. There are many other health professionals who can look at your overall health and guide you in the process of healing rosacea: naturopaths, functional-medicine practitioners or/and holistic nutritionists.

- Remember that every piece of great advice, hint, or knowledge won't make any difference until you put it into practice. In the end, only you have the power to heal your skin.

Good luck!

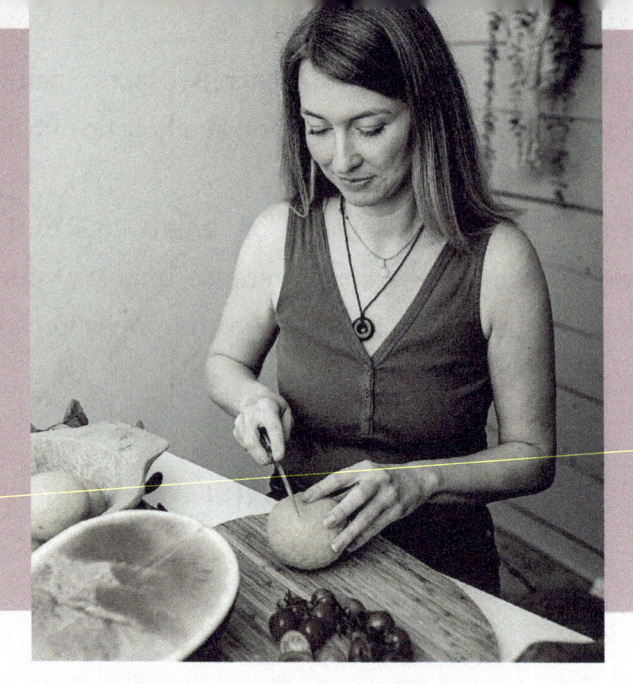

Thank You

For purchasing this book, supporting my work and passion for holistic wellness. I hope you have learnt something about rosacea and natural ways of bringing balance back to your body, and I have inspired you to nurture your health.

I would really appreciate it if you leave a short and honest review for this book on Amazon. This helps to make the book more visible to other rosacea sufferers and would help them to make a conscious choice about whether this publication is suitable for them.

If you have any questions, you can contact me through my Instagram profile. Please follow my account for motivation and tips on healing rosacea.

alicia.piot

Alicia Piot

RESOURCES AND REFERENCES:

Websites:

Link between rosacea and systemic inflammatory diseases (dermatologytimes.com)

Rosacea: Symptoms, Causes, and Management - DermNet (dermnetnz.org)

Possible Root Causes Of Rosacea And How To Treat Them Naturally (rupahealth.com)

Functional Medicine Treatments For Inflammation - Foods & Supplements (richmondfunctionalmedicine.com)

Books:

- "Chronic Inflammation" – Sashwati Roy
- "Inflammation – The Source of Chronic Disease: How To Treat it with Herbs And Natural Healing" – Christine Herbert
- "Holistic Rx : Your Guide to Healing Chronic Inflammation and Disease" – Madiha Saeed
- "The Complete Anti-Inflammatory Diet Cookbook for Beginners: 600 Easy Anti-inflammatory Recipes with 21-Day Meal Plan to Reduce Inflammation" – Fernando K. Rankin
- "Anti-Inflammatory Diet" – LR Smith
- "The Anti-Inflammatory Diet & Action Plans: 4-Week Meal Plans to Heal the Immune System and Restore Overall Health" – Dorothy Calimeris

- "The Anti-inflammatory Kitchen Cookbook" – Leslie Langevin
- "The Autoimmune Answer: Using Functional Medicine to address the cause, eliminate symptoms, and optimize quality of life" – Dr John Bartemus

Podcasts (found on Spotify):

Treating Adult Acne & Rosacea form the Inside Out with Dr Todd LePine

Resolving Acne, Psoriasis, and Other Skin Issues Using Functional Medicine

The Gut-Skin Connection – Leaky Gut, Rosacea, Acne, Eczema, Keratosis Pilaris & Psoriasis

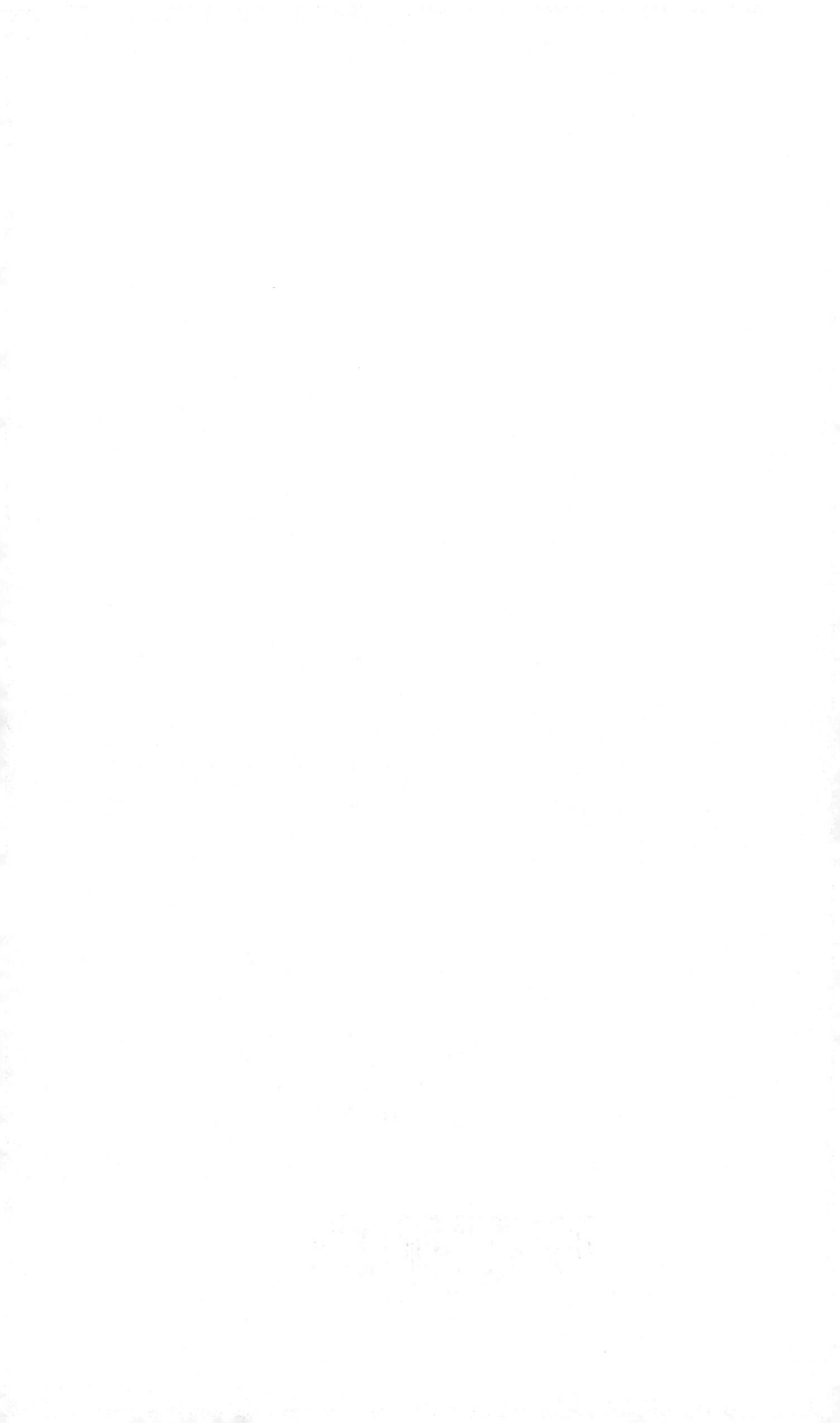

Made in the USA
Monee, IL
21 December 2023